MENOPAUSE

NO NEED TO PANIC

ODILE BAGOT
Doctor of Gynecology

FIREFLY BOOKS

Table of Contents

Introduction

Menopause is nothing to fear! I've gone through it myself, and I'm a content woman in my sixties. So let's explore this turning point in life together and find out what might, and might not, happen to you. At least you'll know what to expect, right?

First and foremost, menopause is different for each woman, since there are as many ways to experience menopause as there are women. However, there is no need to panic — there is a solution for every symptom! The transition to menopause marks a midpoint in life, and it's also an opportunity to reflect back on our life experiences and look forward with determination to a future where you will be even more actively involved. To do this, you will need to take care of your body. Since you will be needing it for a few more decades, you might as well keep it in shape!

Wouldn't you like greater peace of mind and perhaps less negativity in your social and family interactions and friendships, including in your love life? This guide will provide you with valuable advice to support you through this process, body and soul.

What Is Menopause, Exactly?

▌ A Biological Process ▌

Before we get into the nitty-gritty, we first need to agree on what menopause is: It is, simply put, the period in a woman's life when menstruation and the ovarian function end for good.

The somewhat rocky phase that precedes menopause is called perimenopause. A woman is only considered to be in menopause when she has not had a period for a full year. You likely have tons of questions already, right?

How many women are affected? Why does menstruation stop? At what age does it usually stop? How can you be sure you're menopausal? And, most importantly, what are the symptoms?

Menopause Statistics

Nearly
1.3 million American women
start menopause every year, so you are not alone!

It is estimated that
85%
of postmenopausal women have experienced a symptom associated with menopause.

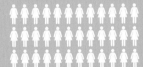

It is estimated that
1.2 billion women
worldwide will be menopausal or postmenopausal by 2030.

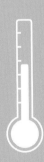

Three out of four women
experience hot flashes.

The median age women begin menopause is
51 years
and initial symptoms start at
47 years.

Menopause symptoms last an average of
four to eight years.

From the Latin *Menopausis*, menopause means the end of menstrual periods. At birth, the ovaries have a predefined supply of ovarian follicles, which are sacs that contain eggs. During puberty, the hypothalamus, which is located at the base of the brain, sends a signal that triggers ovulation, resulting in the release of an egg from a follicle every month. The supply of eggs is limited, however, and menopause begins once the supply of eggs is depleted.

Menopause occurs when your ovaries run out of eggs!

As the egg matures, the follicle secretes estrogen and then, in the second part of the cycle, progesterone. When her progesterone level declines, a woman gets her period.

If pregnancy occurs, the follicle becomes the corpus luteum, which ensures the development of the embryo until the trophoblast, which will develop into the placenta, takes over. At the start of a woman's menstrual cycle, the pituitary gland secretes two hormones — FSH (follicle-stimulating hormone) and LH (luteinizing hormone) — that regulate the recruitment of a primordial follice and its maturation and trigger ovulation. FSH stimulates the growth of the follicle, which contains the egg. When it is mature, LH gives the go-ahead for ovulation. The menstrual cycle is a finely tuned system regulated by the interaction between the ovarian hormones (estradiol and progesterone) and the pituitary hormones. When the number of follicles decreases and, consequently, the levels of hormones decrease as well, FSH increases. This is what happens during menopause.

As we get closer to menopause, and the follicular reserve becomes ever more depleted, the intrinsic quality of the eggs diminishes. This is why, from a certain age, it is no longer possible to become pregnant even if ovulation is still occuring. The end of follicular activity is mainly genetically determined. However, it also depends on environmental conditions. Smoking, for example, hastens menopause, on average, by two years, and chemotherapy can accelerate it by several years. When the follicular reserves start to dwindle, periods become irregular. This phase is called perimenopause. Once the reserve is fully depleted, estrogen and progesterone plummet, FSH goes through the roof, and you're in menopause!

The ovaries have two functions:

- **Exocrine** — directed toward the outside of the body and marked by the monthly release of the egg.

- **Endocrine** — directed internally, via the secretion of the two main hormones in women, which are estrogen and progesterone.

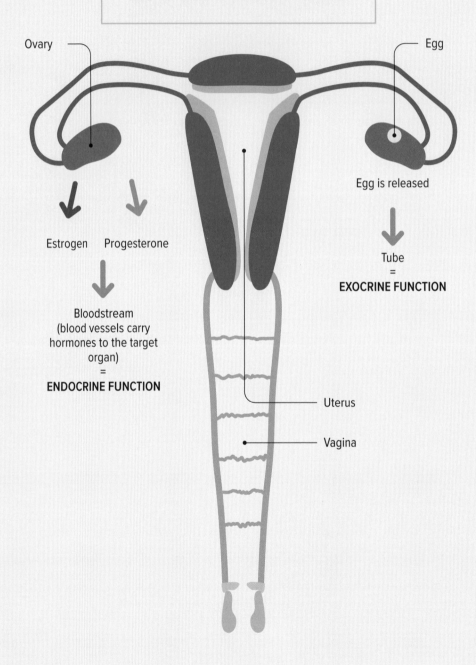

How the Ovaries Work

Ovary

Egg

Egg is released

Estrogen   Progesterone

Tube
=
EXOCRINE FUNCTION

Bloodstream
(blood vessels carry
hormones to the target
organ)
=
ENDOCRINE FUNCTION

Uterus

Vagina

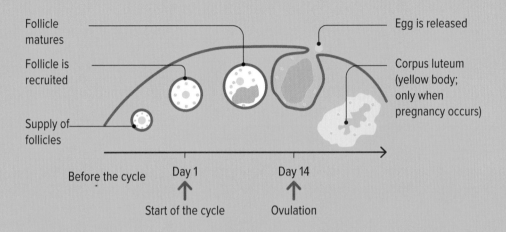

Exocrine Function

Follicle matures

Follicle is recruited

Supply of follicles

Egg is released

Corpus luteum (yellow body; only when pregnancy occurs)

Before the cycle

Day 1
↑
Start of the cycle

Day 14
↑
Ovulation

Endocrine Function

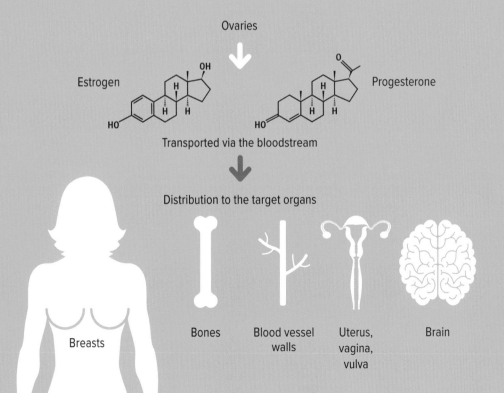

Ovaries

Estrogen

Progesterone

Transported via the bloodstream

Distribution to the target organs

Breasts

Bones

Blood vessel walls

Uterus, vagina, vulva

Brain

▮ At What Age Does It Happen? ▮

Menopause generally begins between the ages of 45 and 55 years. On average, 83 percent of women between the ages of 50 and 54 years are menopausal.

Since the average age for the onset of menopause for women in the United States

> **The average age for the onset of menopause is 51 years.**

is about 51 years and that life expectancy is about 81 years, we can deduce that menopause/postmenopause lasts a good 30 years. This is a significant amount of time so it's certainly worthwhile to find out more about it!

When menopause occurs before the age of 40, it is called premature menopause or, more specifically, premature ovarian insufficiency (POI). Quite fortunately, it is a rare condition and is often genetic. When menopause happens between 40 and 45 years of age, it is called early menopause.

Hormonal treatment is essential in cases of premature menopause, as the risk of osteoporosis and stroke increases very significantly. Women who experience early menopause are advised to undergo a cardiovascular and bone assessment, to help ensure they don't suffer any ill effects due to their lack of hormones. Menopause past the age of 55 is generally considered to be late menopause. Late menopause has not been linked to cardiovascular or bone-related concerns, but it can be associated with an increased risk of breast and uterine cancers, particularly among women who are overweight.

Estrogen and Menopause

Before menopause
(period of genital activity, regular cycles)

Ovulation

Period

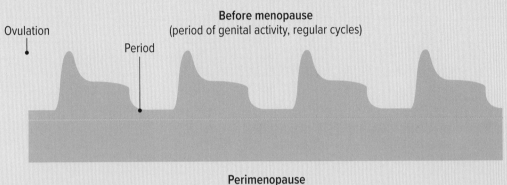

Perimenopause

Normal cycle

Period

Breast tenderness

Abnormal bleeding

Normal cycle

Period

Hot flashes

No period

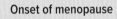

Onset of menopause

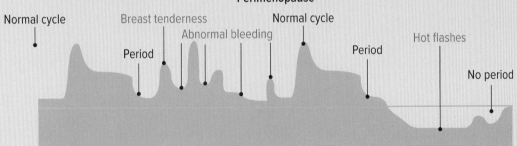

Deep menopause

Estrogen levels and fluctuations   Estradiol threshold of 25 pg/ml

▌The Diagnosis ▌

Although menopause is not considered to be a condition, it is characterized by a number of clinical and biological signs.

If it has been at least a year since your last period and you are around 50 years of age or older, you are very likely in

There is no reliable test to confirm menopause.

menopause. There are, however, always exceptions to the rule. For instance, before the age of 50, even after a year of amenorrhea (no periods), an ovulation cycle can occur in 10 percent of women.[1] Before that fateful year without menstruating, most women are impatiently wondering where they are in all this. Unfortunately, there is no reliable biological test to confirm or rule out menopause. The level of follicle-stimulating hormone (FSH) produced by the pituitary gland increases as we approach menopause, but this is not a sufficient indicator on its own to diagnose menopause. At most, being over the age of 50 and having an FSH level above 25 IU/L indicates you may not need to use birth control, even if you have had a period within the past year.

Testing the progesterone level is more interesting. A progesterone-only pill can be given for 10 days to see if menstruation starts up after treatment is stopped. The sequence is repeated over the next three months if menstruation has not occurred. If the woman has not had a period after this, she is likely in menopause.

1. Sally C. Curtin, Joyce C. Abma, and Kathryn Kost, *2010 Pregnancy Rates Among U.S. Women*, NCHS health e-stat, 2015.

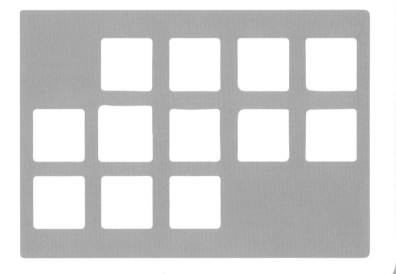

Quick tip:
1 year without a period after the age of **50**
= menopause!

▮ The Symptoms ▮

Some 85 percent of women experience at least one symptom in addition to the end of menstruation, and as many as 20 to 25 percent report a change in their quality of life. Menopause is characterized by two types of events: what can be seen or experienced and what happens completely unnoticed...

What You Will Experience

Hot Flashes

Those dreaded hot flashes! Almost impossible to escape, they often go hand in hand with menopause and can last for a varied amount of time, depending on the woman. Some women don't have them at all, while others can experience them for a number of years.

> **Very few fortunate women do not have any hot flashes!**

Genitourinary Syndrome of Menopause (GSM)

Vaginal dryness and a fickle bladder sometimes develop slightly later in life (generally two or three years after menopause, but it differs from woman to woman, and some women do not experience this at all!).

Mood and sleep disturbances as well as joint pain are also common complaints. "It sucks," as your kids might say!

What Can Go Unnoticed

We need to keep in mind that osteoporosis and stroke can sneak up on us later in life. You might not experience any symptoms of these diseases until they become critical, so it's best to discuss with your health-care provider. At this point, you are no doubt wondering why the title of this guide is *Menopause, No Need to Panic.* Because you're getting a bit worked up right?

There is, however, no need for concern. This guide will explain everything to you, without drama, and you will get advice about how to stay happy and positive and, above all, maintain good health while going through this stage in your life... Yay! But before we discuss menopause further, we first need to have a little chat about perimenopause.

Menopause Symptoms

Brain
- Trouble with memory, concentration and sleeping
- Increased risk of depression
- Mood problems

Face
- Hot flashes

Heart and blood vessels
- Increased risk of cardiovascular disease (since arteries are no longer as well protected)

Stomach
- Weight gain
- Redistribution of fat (especially in the abdominal area)

Bladder
- Increased sensitivity
- Risk of incontinence

Vagina
- Vaginal dryness
- Fragile vaginal mucosa
- Sexual difficulties
- Greater risk of infection

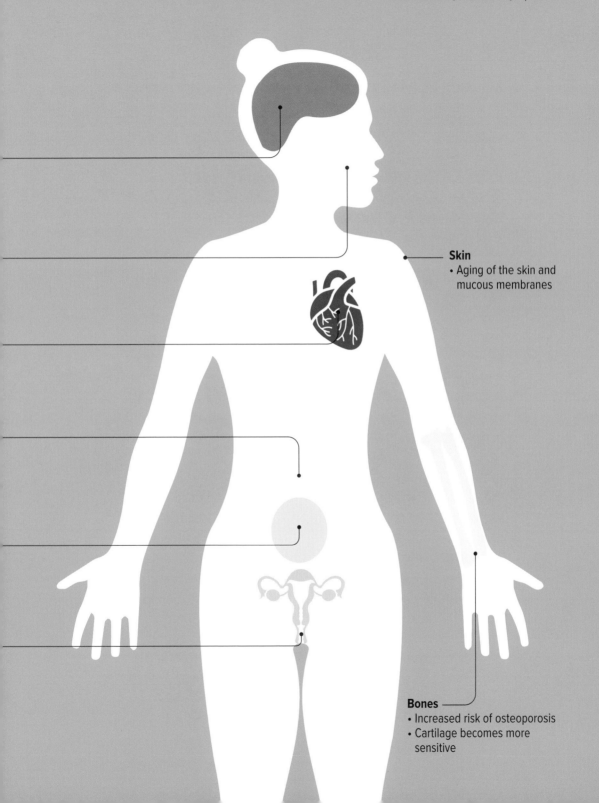

Skin
- Aging of the skin and mucous membranes

Bones
- Increased risk of osteoporosis
- Cartilage becomes more sensitive

Perimenopause

How Does It Develop?

Although it is fairly easy to define menopause, perimenopause is a bit more fuzzy. When does it start? How long does it last? What exactly happens? Is there still a possibility of becoming pregnant?

The average age perimenopause begins is 45 and a half, and it can last from three to eight years. Since this is a serious publication, dear readers, I will share the World Health Organization definition. They define it as "the period immediately prior to the menopause (when the endocrinological, biological and clinical features of approaching menopause commence) and the first year after the menopause." All of these signs indicating that menopause is around the corner are, unfortunately, the consequences of the ovaries getting older. During perimenopause, the ovaries' exocrine and endocrine functions (i.e., the eggs they produce and the hormones they secrete) begin to change. The last remaining eggs, which are close to their "best before" date, are less fertile. Moreover, our hormones have gone rogue, and the important balance between estrogen and progesterone is off kilter. So there is the cause of all of these problems!

> The average age perimenopause begins is 45 and a half years.

The Delicate Balance Between Estrogen and Progesterone

Imagine having the relative weights of these two hormones balancing on each side of a scale. When the balance is maintained, cycles are regular and periods last a week and are not too heavy or preceded by premenstrual syndrome, such as mood swings and breast pain.

During perimenopause, things can become a bit topsy-turvy: You can experience unexpected hormonal swings and, without any warning, your ovaries can take you through a period of estrogen deficiency to disproportionate progesterone production.

If ovulation is on stand-by for a few weeks or months, your hormones will be at their lowest levels. Low estrogen levels are why you experience hot flashes, mood swings, low energy and have trouble sleeping. Basically, it's a menopause preview.

Even if only progesterone production is affected, either in terms of the amount in general or cyclical fluctuations, you will have a relative excess of estrogen, which means problems with your cycle, menorrhagia (very heavy periods), metrorrhagia (breakthrough bleeding) and, of course, mastodynia (pain and tenderness in the breasts). All these things can also certainly affect your mood!

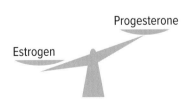

Progesterone

Estrogen

Low progesterone
(which means a relative excess of estrogen)

Low Estrogen

When estrogen levels are low, the ovaries go into a temporary hibernation, which leads to, as we've seen, hot flashes, mood swings and sleep problems.

Hormonal Therapy

During this temporary phase of low estrogen, it is too early to be prescribed menopausal hormone therapy (MHT), also called hormone replacement therapy (HRT), since ovulation could suddenly start up again. And if, all of a sudden, you think that your hot flashes are subsiding, don't forget to pack some sanitary products if you go away on vacation — your monthly visitor could very well tag along! And if the hot flashes persist after you've exhausted all other solutions and you can't deal with them any more, you may be prescribed hormone therapy before the required one year without menstruation. Your doctor may prescribe an appropriate dose of progesterone to stop ovulation and add a low dose of estrogen to help. Hormone therapy for menopause is different because it involves a progestin (synthetic progesterone) that is biologically similar but that cannot stop ovulation during perimenopause.

> During this time, your monthly visitor could very well tag along!

Nonhormonal Therapy

Since there is currently a tendency to demonize hormones (often unfairly), many women are looking for alternative treatment options. Throughout this guide, you will be provided with specific indications for homeopathic treatments, which, as the word "treatment" implies, are medicinal products that must meet particular standards to be commercially available, even if a prescription is not required. In the United States, natural remedies and dietary supplements are overseen by the federal Food and Drug Administration. However, unlike medicines, natural remedies do not require FDA approval. Supplement companies must simply provide evidence that their products are safe and that their label claims are truthful and not misleading. In Canada, natural health products are regulated by Health Canada. Readers are advised to always speak with their health care provider before beginning any treatment. A doctor may recommend these homeopathic treatments or other natural health remedies, and they may even be cov-

You have a lot of choices beyond hormones. Find out more!

ered by your healthcare plan. For example, acupuncture is a treatment option you may want to consider and is available from many accredited practitioners.

And to be thorough, I also discuss phytotherapy (herbal medicine), dietary supplements and aromatherapy (essential oils) in this section. Essential oils have powerful pharmacological properties and, therefore, should be used with caution.

To counter the effects of low estrogen levels, which can lead to hot flashes and mood problems, the following homeopathic treatments may be helpful:

• **Sepia officinalis** for depressed mood.

• **Lachesis mutus** for irritability and intense hot flashes.

In aromatherapy, clary sage is the essential oil generally used to help alleviate menopausal symptoms. Essential oils that behave similarly to estrogen (e.g., sage, anise, fennel, celery, ravensara, anise, hops) should not be used by women with certain gynecological conditions, such as breast cancer or symptomatic fibroids.

A number of dietary supplements that are specifically designed for perimenopause are also available, but these can differ greatly from one to the next. For example, many of these supplements, such as Omega 3, flax, lupulin, selenium, pollen, Vitamin E or magnesium, can have varied compositions, so you cannot necessarily compare their effectiveness. Women with breast cancer should not, however, take food supplements that contain soya.

Important note!
Some essential oils and dietary supplements are contraindicated for women with breast cancer.

Helpful Dietary Supplements

Selenium

Flaxseed and flax oil

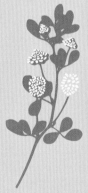

Pollen

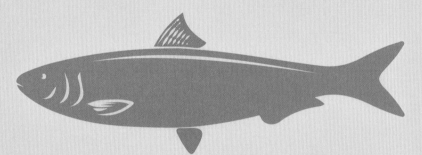

Omega 3

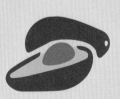

Vitamin E

Magnesium

Lupulin

Low Progesterone

When the balance between estrogen and progesterone is off, the higher estrogen level can produce the following:

- short cycles, with periods closer together;
- longer-lasting periods with heavy bleeding;
- premenstrual syndrome.

Premenstrual Syndrome and Irregular Cycles

Many women experience premenstrual syndrome a few days before getting their period. It is often associated with breast tenderness, water retention and mood changes.

> You can track your periods in a menstrual journal.

There can be pelvic pain, migraines and acne, although those symptoms are rare. If you miss your period for a few months, even if you have hot flashes, it will likely have little impact on your health.

The alternative — bleeding every two weeks — is no picnic either. To help you make sense of your cycles, you can keep a menstrual journal, where you can write down the date when you get your period, the type of flow and any unusual bleeding. To assess your blood loss, your health-care provider may order a blood test to check your hemoglobin level and your body's iron stores through a ferritin blood test. If necessary, you will need to take an iron supplement, generally in pill form.

In the event of severe anemia, you may need to have an iron infusion. Dietary supplements are generally not sufficient to resolve seriously low levels of iron, since iron is poorly absorbed in the GI tract. As a preventative step, you can get iron essentially by eating red meat, but you have to like the less-desirable cuts, such as the organs.

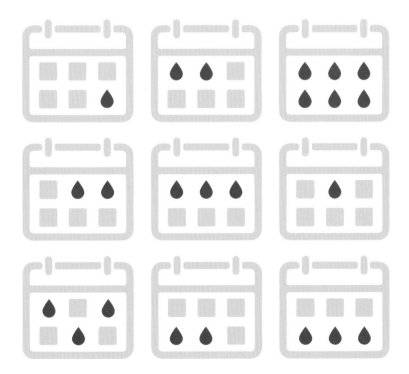

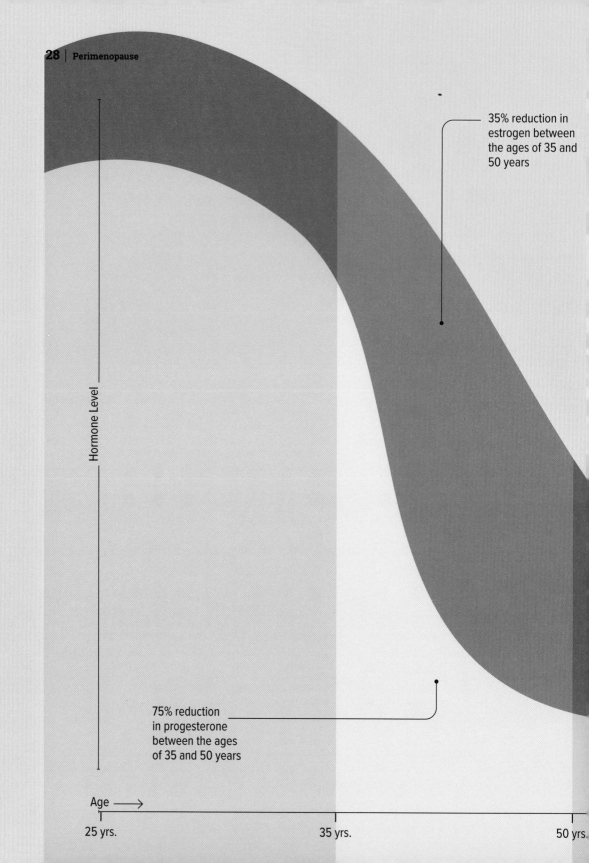

35% reduction in estrogen between the ages of 35 and 50 years

Hormone Level

75% reduction in progesterone between the ages of 35 and 50 years

Age ⟶

25 yrs.

35 yrs.

50 yrs.

Estrogen and Progesterone Levels

Estrogen

Progesterone

60 yrs.   75 yrs.

Treatments

Since there is no available drug that can lower estrogen levels, you may be given progestin as an "antidote." There are two ways to take progestin-based pills:

• **Intermittently**, from day 5, 10 or 15 of your cycle, up to day 25, to improve premenstrual syndrome and normalize your cycle.

• **Continuously**, to block your cycle so you are in amenorrhea (no periods).

Quick tip: the first day of your cycle is the first day of your period.

Two types of drugs are used to offset low estrogen levels, a biologically similar progesterone that is well tolerated but not sufficient to prevent ovulation, and thereby be used as contraception. Antigonadotropic progesterone is the other drug.

The same result can be achieved with a progestin-only IUD, which acts specifically on the uterus (and does not interfere with a woman's cycle or hormone fluctuations) to reduce the thickness of the endometrial lining. A thinner lining means less bleeding. This can be a great solution for women who still get their periods and are concerned about (or don't tolerate) systemic hormones. The progestin in this type of IUD more or less delivers the product locally, with minimal passage into the bloodstream.

To make your cycles more regular, homeopathic treatments could involve folliculinum or luteinum. Ask your homeopathic doctor for the specific product that's best for you.

In aromatherapy, chaste-berry (or chaste tree) essential oil is generally used to help correct cycles, since it has a similar action to progesterone.

Hormonal Ups and Downs

All of these hormone fluctuations can certainly affect your mood. Many women, especially if they have full lives, with family, social engagements and careers, feel more sensitive and irritable before their period. Others may have a rockier experience and not feel like themselves — the slightest thing can set them off. These women may find that something that didn't bother them at all before suddenly feels like a complete disaster.

This hormonal yo-yoing can be exhausting and often leads to depression. Don't be shy about seeing your doctor to find out more.

Your lifestyle habits, physical activity and diet can also affect your hormone fluctuations. Moreover, extra pounds can quickly add up... but that's another story!

Take it seriously if you're feeling depressed, and talk to your doctor!

Contraception and Fertility

If you want to have a child and you're over 45, your chances of getting pregnant are slim. Aside from a donated egg and surrogate, there is no medically assisted reproduction technique that can help a woman whose ovaries are no longer producing eggs. However, even at this age, you should not take any risks. You absolutely should be using birth control!

Birth Control Methods

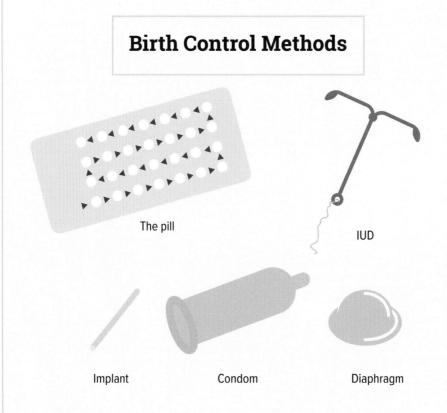

The pill

IUD

Implant

Condom

Diaphragm

Which Type of Birth Control Should You Choose?

The Pill and the Implant

Certain birth control methods should not be used by women over 45 years of age, starting with the pill, which may have been your trusted companion for a long time. "The pill" generally refers to a combination of synthetic progesterone and estrogen. The ethinyl estradiol estrogen that most pills contain is particularly toxic for the cardiovascular system. Since there's no escaping our ageing arteries, the pill and blood vessels are generally not a good match after 40: You are at risk for phlebitis, pulmonary embolisms, strokes and myocardial infarctions. Not fun at all!

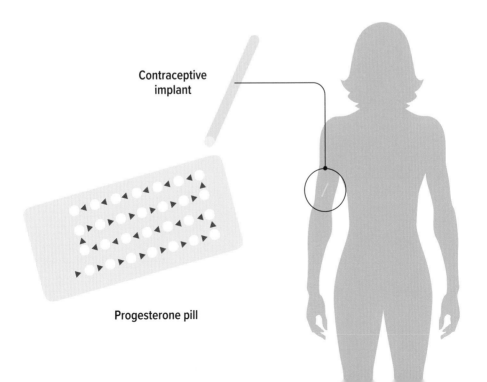

Contraceptive implant

Progesterone pill

If you truly don't want to give up the pill, you may be able to stay on it as long as you have absolutely no risk factors other than age: you don't smoke, don't have high blood pressure, are not overweight, don't have high cholesterol and don't have a family history of cardiovascular disease.

There is also a progestin-only pill, without added estrogen. It's generally called the minipill or POP. These products are effective and generally well tolerated, outside of possible spotting (slight bleeding for a few days to a few weeks). There is no major cardiovascular contraindication when prescribing these products. It's a good compromise if you have been a fan of the pill for a long time or if you don't like the idea of having a foreign object inserted in your body, such as an IUD.

These pills work by changing the mucus produced by the cervix, slowing the movement of sperm through the uterus. Since fertility drops during perimenopause, the effectiveness of the minipill can be sufficient, but you still need to remember to take your pill every day, at about the same time (within a few hours).

Another progestin-only option is an implant such as Nexplanon. It is certainly an effective form of birth control, but you may wonder how necessary this really is after the age of 45, when fertility is so low? Additionally, your menstrual cycle can become unpredictable. About one-third of women do not have periods, which is great; about one-third have occasional bleeding, which is fine; and about one-third have bleeding all the time, which is a nightmare!

Intrauterine Device (IUD)

If you prefer an IUD, there are progestin-only (Mirena and Kyleena) and copper options. Even though the progestin versions can be considered "hormonal" contraception, all IUD are categorized as barrier methods. In fact, the minimal flow of hormones in the blood interferes very little with the menstrual cycle. Progestin simply thickens the cervical mucus to prevent sperm from entering the uterus. And as an added bonus, since progestin is continuously released in the endometrium, you may stop having your periods completely with Mirena and menstrual bleeding decreases significantly with Kyleena, and that's not a bad thing in perimenopause!

Copper IUDs, on the other hand, tend to result in heavier bleeding during periods. In certain situations, where there are definite hormone contra-indications, such as breast cancer or if your periods are naturally light, a copper IUD may be an option. It is not, however, an option if you have excessive bleeding or fibroids.

The choice between the two types of IUDs is truly a case-by-case decision. Discuss with your gynecologist or other health-care provider, and you may even consider testing one and then the other!

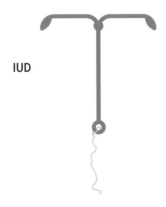

IUD

Other methods

Spermicides are fine and provide quite adequate birth control during perimenopause. The good old condom is also always an appropriate option. And lastly, there is another radical option: permanent birth control through a tubal ligation procedure (surgical sterilization).

You can use a condom or diaphragm with spermicide.

This procedure requires laparoscopy (insertion of an instrument via the abdominal wall) and general anesthesia. This may be a bit too much to consider for someone approaching menopause. However, it's not easy to completely rule out the option of ever conceiving again, even if, logically, you're certain about not wanting any more children. For this reason, you need to take the time to carefully consider this option (some jurisdictions have a mandatory waiting period for any irreversible procedure).

Tubal Ligation

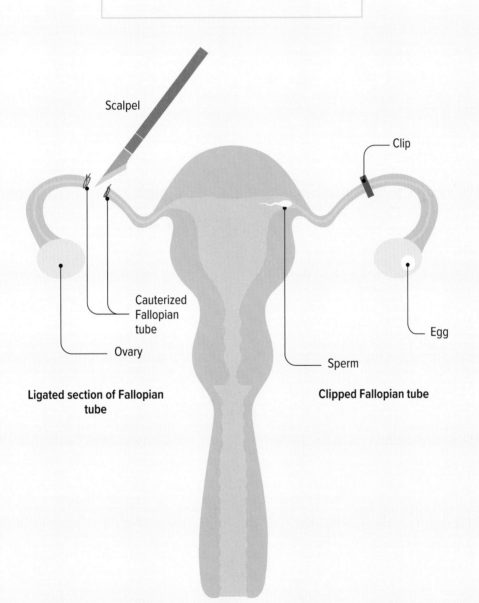

Scalpel

Clip

Cauterized
Fallopian
tube

Ovary

Egg

Sperm

**Ligated section of Fallopian
tube**

Clipped Fallopian tube

How Do You Know if You Can Still Conceive?

Once you are over the age of 50 and have gone a year without menstruating (or two years after the age of 48), there is no question: Baby-making is definitely a thing of the past. Before then, however, how do you know if you can still conceive? It is

> **After the age of 50, if FSH is above 25 mIU/ml, it is not possible to conceive.**

done by testing for levels of follicle-stimulating hormone (FSH), which is the hormone produced by the pituitary gland to signal the development of a follicle, subsequently resulting in ovulation. Levels are expressed in milli-international units per milliliters (mIU/ml).

FSH levels increase progressively starting around the age of 40, and once you hit menopause, they remain very high. After the age of 50, if FSH is above 25 mIU/ml, it is not possible to conceive, even if you are still having periods.

This is particularly helpful to know if your birth control method has stopped your periods. Can you stop taking your pill? Can your IUD be taken out for good? In terms of pregnancy risk, the answer is simple: When the FSH level is above 25 mIU/ml after 50 years of age, there is zero risk of pregnancy. And what about your periods? If your FSH level is still hovering close to 25 mIU/ml and you don't have any hot flashes, you could very well start menstruating again after removing your IUD or stopping the pill. The choice is yours, but it's certainly convenient to be rid of it all! If your FSH is quite high (above 45 mIU/ml), you may decide to take your chances and stop using birth control.

Menopause Has Arrived!

▌ How Does It Happen? ▌

Have you turned 50? Has it been more than a year since your last period? Have you given up your tampons, cups or other period products? You are definitely in menopause!

Women between the ages of 45 and 50, however, need to wait two years from their last period before popping the champagne. You know that, despite the hearsay and other stress-inducing chatter, it's time to party! No more "off" weeks because of your period, no more painful breasts, no more premenstrual syndrome! And of course, no more concerns about birth control — you can go wild without the risk of pregnancy! But don't forget about sexually transmitted infections; they don't go away with menopause...

However, for most women, the onset of menopause is also accompanied by symptoms that are not always pleasant, such as climacteric symptoms.

These include vasomotor instabilities (also referred to as hot flashes), genitourinary syndrome of menopause (GSM, which involves vaginal dryness and bladder issues), and mood and sleep problems. Nothing to do with climate change, "climacteric" (a word not used much anymore) comes from a Greek word that literally means "rung of a ladder" but means a critical point. In our case it refers to problems associated with menopause due to estrogen deficiency. In other words, it's a transition phase marked by the end of the reproductive function, which we will help you get through with a bit of humor!

▮ Vasomotor Instability ▮

These are the most common and characteristic signs of menopause. Few women are spared and they generally report that this phase greatly affects their quality of life. However, there are a number of ways to get through this, or at the very least reduce the impact.

The Mechanism

Why do menopausal women have hot flashes? Even the most recent research has failed to unlock the key to this mystery! The body's temperature regulation system, your internal thermostat, is located in the brain, more specifically the hypothalamus. Before menopause, it is set to detect temperature fluctuations of 0.7°F (0.4°C), called the neutral temperature threshold. In other words, when your body temperature fluctuates more than 0.7°F (0.4°C), the body releases this excess heat as sweat or by dilating the skin's blood vessels in order to cool down.

A menopausal woman experiencing hot flashes has a neutral temperature threshold of close to zero, so her cooling system kicks in at the drop of a hat!

Estrogen also has an important role in hot flashes. The numbers themselves are not so much what matters. What's critical is how quickly they change. It is, therefore, easy to understand why hot flashes are more frequent at the start of menopause, when hormones are all over the place, than further into menopause, when estrogen levels simply plummet.

The Mechanism of Hot Flashes

1

A sudden drop in estrogen disrupts the body's temperature regulation center in the hypothalamus.

2

The hypothalamus responds as it does when the body is overheated. We do not, however, know why or how estrogen levels affect the hypothalamus to such a degree.

3

The brain sends out a signal to cool the body. It tells the heart, blood vessels and nervous system to get rid of the heat.

4

The body attempts to cool itself and produces sweat. The heart beats faster, the blood vessels dilate to get more blood flowing and the sweat glands are activated.

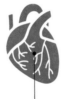

Other reactionary systems are also thought to be involved in hot flashes based on observations of how people have reacted to certain drugs. Most notably, antidepressants that affect serotonin levels diminish hot flashes. It can therefore be surmised that this neurotransmitter plays a part in vasomotor instability. The sympathetic nervous system — the body system that responds to stress (triggering, among other things, a surge in adrenalin and an increase in heart rate, respiratory rate and blood pressure), also triggers hot flashes when stimulated. It could be the mediator between the signal from the hypothalamuses's thermal regulatory center and the peripheral vascular dilation reaction, namely redness and sweating.

Flushing

This term encompasses both dry hot flashes and those accompanied by sweating — the ones more often experienced at night. Dry hot flashes tend to be a daytime occurrence, sometimes followed by a cold, clammy feeling. The perception of flushing is variable. Most often, there is a sensation of heat rising from the chest to the neck and then to the face. Your face may turn red, but it is less noticeable than you would think. Most of the time, the people around you won't notice anything.

Flushing can be accompanied by sweat, with beads of perspiration collecting between the breasts, rising up to the neck and, more rarely, on the face.

The intensity, frequency and tolerance for these episodes also vary greatly, from a few hot spells during the day to waking up fully drenched in the middle of the night with the sheets and your pajamas soaked. They can be triggered by emotion, a warm environment or even spicy foods!

At the start of menopause, more than three-quarters of women will suffer hot flashes to some degree. Five years later, one in two will still be fanning themselves to get relief. I have even seen some very dignified ladies in their 80s asking for a minidose of estrogen to help with hot flashes. Conversely, some lucky women are spared.

Several studies have shown a connection between body mass index (BMI) and hot flashes, with overweight women more prone to them because it's more difficult for their small surface vessels to release heat. The insulating effect of fatty tissue also accounts for the increase in vasomotor instability in women with a higher BMI and more body fat. However, body fat remains a significant source of estrogen, even after menopause, with an excess indicating an increased risk for developing breast and endometrial cancers.

However, while physical activity will help you feel better mentally and physically, it does not, unfortunately, reduce hot flashes.

Estrogen supplementation invariably helps alleviate hot flashes.

Estrogen supplementation invariably helps alleviate hot flashes caused by menopause. If the hot flashes persist, we then look for another reason for the vasomotor instability, such as a thyroid disorder, hypertension or hypoglycemia. Nonetheless, hormonal treatment for menopausal symptoms is not always feasible for all women or even desirable, so nonhormonal alternative treatments may be a solution to the problem

Nonhormonal Treatments

There are all kinds of nonhormonal treatments: chemical; homeopathic; aromatherapy; phytotherapy (i.e., herbal remedies), particularly phytoestrogens, which are compounds that act like natural estrogen.

Antidepressants

Antidepressants that belong to the family known as serotonin reuptake inhibitors can help. Here's how it works:

Serotonin is a thermoregulatory neurotransmitter, so increasing the amount of it in the brain can help manage hot flashes.

Important note: These drugs interfere with the cytochromes involved in the body's metabolization of the breast cancer drug tamoxifen, making it less effective. Two examples of specific serotonin reuptake inhibitors with this effect are paroxetine (Paxil and Pexeva) and fluoxetine (Prozac).

> Some antidepressants reduce hot flashes but can interfere with breast cancer treatment.

Beta-alanine

Beta-alanine is an amino acid. It is thought to interact with the peripheral mechanism associated with hot flashes at the vascular level. The daily dosage is one to three tablets. It is not considered to be habit-forming, and there are no precautions for use or associated major side effects.

Homeopathic Remedies

If looking for a homeopathic remedy for hot flashes, you can take a shot in the dark and try Acteane (Boiron) or one of the many other products specially formulated to alleviate symptoms of menopause. As for efficacy, some of these products have, in fact, been tested against a placebo and were shown to have performed slightly better. While the difference may not have been significant, the placebo effect has a response rate of about 50 percent for hot flashes. In the end, however, aren't we simply looking for risk-free relief from such remedies? If you want to adjust and personalize your treatment, it's best to consult a homeopathic doctor who, based on your specific symptoms, may choose products such as *Lachesis mutus*, belladonna, *Sanguinaria*

> **You might want to consider trying homeopathic remedies to see if any are right for you.**

canadensis (bloodroot), *Sepia officinalis* or sulfuric acid. One study showed that when homeopathic treatment is individualized, regardless of the clinical situation, its effect exceeds that of a placebo in a statistically significant manner.[2]

2. Mathie, R.T., Lloyd, S.M., Legg, L.A. *et al*. Randomised placebo-controlled trials of individualised homeopathic treatment: systematic review and meta-analysis. *Syst Rev* **3**, 142 (2014). https://doi.org/10.1186/2046-4053-3-142

Aromatherapy

As a remedy for estrogen deficiency and vasomotor instabilities, clary sage is consistently popular. It can be used alone or with other essential oils, such as cypress, green anise or mint. It is administered transdermally by diluting it into a base oil such as apricot kernel oil and massaging the lower abdomen. Clary sage can also be taken orally as long as it is a food-grade product that is safe to consume, by adding two drops to a tablespoon of honey. It can also be inhaled using an essential oil diffuser.

Important note: Essential oils with estrogenic properties are contraindicated for women with breast cancer.

Phytotherapy

Phytotherapy is a herbal remedy practice that is based on science rather than tradition. Over the past 10 years, some 300 natural products and 600 plants have been identified as having estrogen-receptor binding properties. In essence, these substances' molecules resemble estrogen and can therefore "trick" the receptors located on the surface of the target cells (breasts, endometrium, vagina, brain, bones, etc.). The effect can, to varying degrees, be inhibitory (lessen the effect) or excitatory (activate the effect). So here's where things get a bit complicated.

Contrary to its proposed usage, sage's estrogenic activity has not been fully documented. Yams, meanwhile, affect the synthesis of corticosteroids more than the synthesis of the female hormones, i.e., estrogen and progesterone. Since estrogen deficiency is not the sole cause of hot flashes, plants like black cohosh (*Actaea racemosa*) can have an effect via the central thermoregulatory system — in other words, your personal thermostat!

Plants That Can Help Alleviate Symptoms of Menopause

Soy
(beans)

Clover
(leaves)

Alfalfa
(leaves)

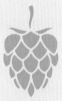

Hops
(cones)

Kudzu
(leaves and root)

Licorice
(root)

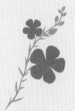

Flax
(seeds)

Fennell
(fruit)

Black cohosh, also called cimicifuga, was traditionally used by Indigenous Americans. Its mode of action to counteract hot flashes is complex. It activates the thermoregulatory center via serotonin. There is, however, controversy about its action on the estrogen receptors, as it appears to be both pro- and anti-estrogenic, depending on the target.

Black cohosh has traditionally been used to treat hot flashes, but its mode of action is complex.

As a precautionary measure, the use of *Actaea racemosa* as a herbal remedy (but not as a homeopathic dilution) is contraindicated in gynecological cancers, particularly breast cancer.

Important note: Black cohosh is hepatotoxic, meaning it can harm the liver. It is therefore important to follow the dose instructions.

It is impossible to list all of the herbal remedies on the market that claim to help alleviate symptoms associated with menopause and even less possible to compare them. A number of studies have, however, looked at phytoestrogens, investigating their indications, efficacy, side effects and risks.

Black Cohosh
(all forms)

Contains 1 mg of active ingredient

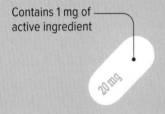

Standardized extract
Dose: one or two per day
Reference product in most studies:
Remifemin

Contains 60% ethanol in a 1:10 ratio

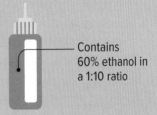

Tincture
Dose: 1/8 to 1/2 teaspoon (0.5–2 ml) per day
diluted in water

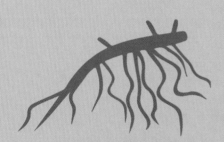

Dried rhizome and roots
Dose: 40 mg per day

Infusion
Root and rhizome: 40 mg in 1/3 cup (150 ml) of
boiling water, strain and drink

With thanks to Jean-Yves Dionne for the indications noted here, from his
article on the Passeport Santé website.

Phytoestrogens

Isoflavones, primarily daidzein and genistein, are the active substances in phytoestrogens. Like black cohosh, their effect is variable and depends on the hormone receptor they act on, thereby triggering both pro- and anti-estrogenic

> **Isoflavones are the active substances in phytoestrogens.**

effects. The transformation of isoflavones into their active compound, equol, depends on the person's intestinal flora. Competent bacteria (i.e., bacteria that can be transformed) are only present in less than half of Western women; conversely, all Asian women have them. In countries like Japan, where soy is prevalent in the diet, women are far less prone to hot flashes because the composition of their intestinal flora has adapted.

The efficacy of the phytoestrogen found in soy is 15 percent higher than a placebo, and the placebo effect is known to reduce hot flashes in one out of two women.

Important note: Because of their estrogenic pharmacological action, phytoestrogens are contraindicated for women with breast or endometrial cancer.

However, this does not necessarily mean that the consumption of soy or soy-based nutritional supplements increases the risk of breast cancer.

Diet

The main estrogenic compounds found in many foods are isoflavones and lignans. In Western countries, lignans account for approximately 80 percent of the population's intake of phytoestrogen, and isoflavones account for the other 20 percent. The proportion varies in vegetarians and individuals whose regular diet includes soy (as a substitute for dairy or meat, for example). A balanced diet rich in vegetables, grains and legumes, along with coffee and tea, is a good source of lignans, so why not make changes to your diet to help alleviate your hot flashes? We still have a way to go to catch up to Japan, where a woman's average daily isoflavone consumption is 45 mg versus 0.4 mg in the West — 100 times less! Bearing in mind that the average isoflavone content

Why not make changes to your diet to help with your hot flashes?

in a soy-based dessert is 44 mg, some diets that replace all dairy products with soy risk an intake that's 10 to 100 times higher than the Asian diet. So tread lightly!

Foods That Contain Isoflavones or Lignans

Isoflavones

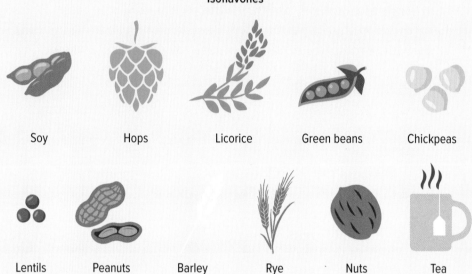

Soy   Hops   Licorice   Green beans   Chickpeas

Lentils   Peanuts   Barley   Rye   Nuts   Tea

Lignans

Seeds (flax, sunflower, rye, sesame, pumpkin)   Whole grains   Fruit (cherries, apples, pears)   Vegetables (carrots, fennel, onion, garlic, celery)   Tea and coffee

Nutritional Supplements

In 2003, a French agency identified over 50 isoflavone-based food supplements that claimed to eliminate virtually all menopause problems.[3] It is certainly a large and profitable market, so the consumer needs to make an effort to stay informed.

The daily dose of an isoflavone supplement should not exceed 40 mg. We are only discussing isoflavones here and not lignans, another major source of phytoestrogens. We need to be careful when a product contains a phytoestrogen from another family, such as lignans (found in hops) or coumestrol (found in alfalfa), in combination with soy, which is also a rich source of isoflavones. We now better understand why it is important for women with breast or uterine cancer to avoid these types of supplements.

(Isoflavones also compete with the breast cancer drug tamoxifen, so they are doubly contraindicated for breast cancer patients who are receiving that drug.) Moreover, given that phytoestrogens interact with the production of thyroid hormones, it is strongly advised people with hypothyroidism (low thyroid) avoid phytoestrogen supplements and limit their dietary intake.

> **Important note: Isoflavones interact with thyroid hormones.**

To conclude, too much overlap is overkill when it comes to phytoestrogens. Do not combine soy-rich foods with dietary supplements and consider your phytoestrogen intake from other sources in your diet.

3. Isabelle Berta-Vanrullen, *Sécurité et bénéfices des phyto-estrogènes apportés par l'alimentation – Recommandations*, Agence française de sécurité sanitaire des aliments, March 2005.

Hormones

If you have tried all the remedies mentioned and hot flashes continue to make your life miserable, especially your nights, menopausal hormone treatment (MHT), also called hormone replacement therapy (HRT) could provide real relief. In fact, the main indication for MHT is treatment of vasomotor instabilities. You will start to feel the effects within two weeks. If hot flashes still bother you after this time, the estrogen dose can be increased, provided your breasts don't become painful or tender. If the thought of hormone treatment concerns you and you still don't know what to believe after all the discussion and debate, go to the last chapter for more information so you can make an informed choice for yourself.

The main indication for MHT is treatment of vasomotor instability.

Adopt a Zen State of Mind

Hot flashes are not a fatal illness and not every woman is affected to the same degree. Everyone experiences menopause differently. Viewing it as a natural life process bringing you toward greater peace of mind will prevent you from seeing every hot flash as a reminder that you are getting older. Think of the hot flash as an old friend who is visiting but has overstayed their welcome and then finally leaves. That might help. Breathe calmly and gently blow out the air upward toward your face.

Elegantly fan yourself with a sheet of paper or discreetly crack open a window. Or simply show everyone your sense of humor and poke fun at yourself by bringing out that beautiful fan you picked up on a trip to Spain and do your best Carmen imitation. Open the window in the middle of the winter and shout out a loud, unabashed "Olé!" to wake up your sleepy colleagues at work!

Relaxation, sophrology (a technique that uses body and mind to create balance and harmony), hypnosis or even mindful meditation are all alternative therapies that can effectively lessen the impact of vasomotor instabilities on your morale and quality of life.

Although physically active women don't have significantly fewer hot flashes than women with a sedentary lifestyle, they often just tend to feel better in their skin, and therefore tend to have a higher tolerance of climacteric (menopausal) symptoms.

Other options are relaxation activities, sophrology, hypnosis and mindful meditation.

If exercise is not your thing, you might enjoy qigong, tai chi, yoga or other activities that combine body awareness, breathing and spirituality.

▮ Genitourinary Syndrome of Menopause ▮

Genitourinary is big word that refers to vaginal dryness and a variety of urinary problems that may accompany menopause. The mucosa in the vulva, vagina, bladder and urethra and even the pelvic floor all require estrogen to remain healthy. When estrogen levels drop drastically, these organs are affected to various degrees.

When Your Bladder Acts Up

The bladder is less able to fight off infections during menopause. It is also more sensitive, less continent and has greater difficulty in managing its contractions (and is therefore said to be "unstable").

Cystitis

During menopause, we see an increase in the number of urinary infections caused by bacteria, such as *Escherichia coli* (*E. coli*). We also see more cases of cystitis, when, although no bacteria are present, all the symptoms indicate cystitis: frequent need to urinate, burning or painful sensation when urinating and a feeling of pressure in the pelvic area.

Urinary Tract Infections

If cystitis is suspected, a urine cytology test is done to detect bacteria. If bacteria is present, it indicates the patient has a urinary tract infection (or UTI). An antibiogram may also be done to check for the bacteria's susceptibility to antibiotics. Currently, a single dose of the urinary antiseptic fosfomycin is prescribed as the first-line treatment. If you have more than four documented infections during a single year, this is called recurrent cystitis. In such cases, a preventative antibiotic may be an option, but a local or systemic estrogen-based therapy is generally the preferred treatment. These have been shown to be effective. MHT is the most common systemic estrogen-based therapy. Local delivery options include ovules (suppositories), vaginal creams and vaginal rings, which release estrogen continuously for three months.

Since the walls of the vagina and the bladder are side by side, the hormone easily passes through the vaginal mucosa to the bladder. Quick tip: apply a small amount of estrogen cream every day at the opening of the urethra (where the urine comes out) to strengthen the urethra's defenses, as this is how germs get in to the bladder.

Vaginally administered estrogen can reduce the frequency of recurrent cystitis.

The four vaginal administration systems

Vaginal ring

Ovule (suppository)

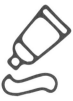

Cream

Single-dose applicator

What Can You Do to Prevent UTIs?

1

Drink plenty of water.

2

Don't hold a full bladder for too long.

3

Urinate after sex.

4

Always wipe yourself from front to back, never the other way around.

5

Avoid sanitary pads and panty liners.

Interstitial Cystitis

Also called painful bladder syndrome, this condition is fortunately rarer and less painful than a UTI. It is, however, much more difficult to treat, since treatment is often not effective, so it can become a chronic problem. It presents as typical cystitis, with bladder discomfort that temporarily feels better after urinating. Paradoxically, a urine culture test does not indicate a bacterial infection (sterile urine) result. In order to accurately diagnose this condition, a cystoscopy (also called a bladder endoscopy) is done.

Antibiotics do nothing to treat interstitial cystitis. When an episode occurs, therapies only treat the symptoms and pain. There are available drug treatments, such as pentosan polysulfate sodium (Elmiron), which produces mixed results. Local estrogen therapy has not shown to be helpful. Long-term management is mainly urological; bladder distention (stretching the bladder with water) and instillation (during which medications are injected into the bladder via a catheter) can help with intense inflammation of the bladder wall. Chronic pain management may require a prescription.

Urinary Problems

Here is a full list of urinary problems that may get worse during menopause. Don't despair, I promise you won't end up in diapers. There are better options available!

Daytime Pollakiuria

This is frequent urination in small amounts during the day. This differs from polyuria, which is increased urination of large volumes caused by taking diuretics or by excessive intake of fluids.

You can help distinguish between these two conditions by keeping a bladder journal (free templates are available online).

Nocturia
The need to urinate at night.

Overactive Bladder
This is an urgent need to urinate, with or without urinary incontinence, combined with pollakiuria and/or nocturia. It is important to identify these problems by discussing with your health-care provider, getting a clinical exam and, sometimes, getting additional tests, such as urodynamic tests, especially when urinary problems are associated

Urgent urination
An overwhelming need to urinate.

Dysuria
Pain or difficulty associated with voiding the bladder.

with urinary incontinence. Available treatment options include local estrogen therapy, medications specifically for the bladder, such as alpha blockers (Toviaz, Ditropan), and exercises to help strengthen the pelvic floor muscles (sometimes referred to as "reeducation").

It's important to adopt proper lifestyle habits: avoid stimulants such as coffee, tea, and cigarettes; drink liquids when you are thirsty but not too much; and don't pee too often, so your bladder maintains its ability to distend.

Don't pee too often so your bladder maintains its ability to distend.

Urinary Incontinence

Urinary incontinence is too often a taboo subject, and we need to talk about it! Talking to your doctor about it is nothing to be embarrassed about, since there are many potential solutions. There are two types of urinary incontinence: stress incontinence (happens when coughing, during physical activity, lifting an item, etc.) and incontinence that happens without warning or immediately after an urge to urinate. More rarely, the reason is a bladder sphincter problem, causing continuous leakage. In any case, the initial step is always reeducation to wake up the bladder's backup muscle, the perineum. For cases of urgent urination with incontinence, alpha blockers can be prescribed. They have varying degrees of success, since their main side effect is dry mouth, which often results in patients discontinuing treatment. People whose incontinence is caused by a prolapsed bladder may be good candidates for surgery, but before undergoing any invasive procedure, urodynamic testing must be done. This involves studying how the bladder and sphincter

> **Talking to your doctor about urinary incontinence is nothing to be embarrassed about.**

respond in various situations that reflect what happens in real life (super full bladder, coughing, trying to stop leakage, etc.). The exam is not painful but there is a bit of discomfort since it involves inserting a catheter into the bladder. If urodynamic testing shows that you indeed have a prolapsed bladder, surgical treatment with placement of bands will completely fix the problem. With age and menopause, everyone has a bladder that tends to droop a bit...

When the Perineum Weakens

The perineum (or pelvic floor), which supports the bladder, vagina and rectum, is affected by the lower estrogen levels during menopause and loses tone over time.

Get to know your pelvic floor! This will help support your bladder, vagina and rectum.

The pelvic muscles therefore tend to drop, which is called prolapse. If the bladder is affected it is called cystocele, and if the rectum is affected it is called rectocele.

Here are a few tips to prevent this:
• Don't carry heavy items.
• Learn how to do hypopressive abdominal exercises.
• Watch your weight.
• Build up your pelvic floor muscles.

You can strengthen your pelvic floor muscles on your own or with a probe and related app, or your healthcare provider may suggest you see a registered pelvic floor therapist. On the positive side of things, you will gain awareness of your pelvic floor, which can lead you to discover many possibilities, including sexual ones.

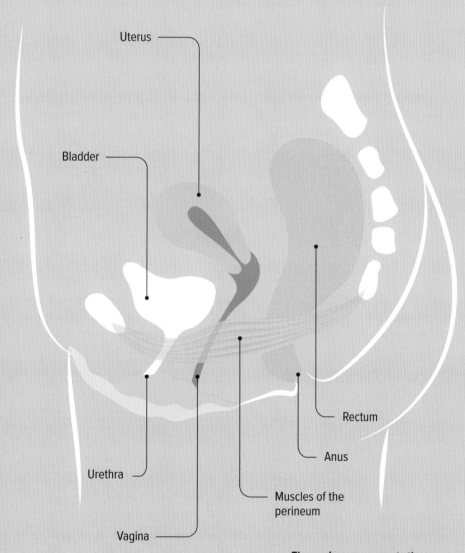

Perineum
(cross section)

Uterus

Bladder

Urethra

Vagina

Muscles of the perineum

Anus

Rectum

The perineum supports the bladder, uterus and rectum.

When You Have Vaginal Dryness

The vagina and vestibule (the part of the vulva between the inside of the labia minora and the opening of the vagina) are naturally moist since they are lined with mucosa and not skin. This mucosa, which depends on hormones, will become thinner and loose elasticity as menopause advances.

Vaginal secretions also decrease, since the lacobacilli component in the flora decreases with the drop in estrogen, which is the bacterium's primary nutrient. Consequently, this means discomfort and sometimes tears during penetration. No need to panic, however, there is also a solution for this!

The Vagina

You may only experience this dryness during sexual intercourse. As with urinary problems, you can take estrogen systemically or locally. You can also take prebiotics or probiotics to help rebuild vaginal flora. A prebiotic provides a nutrient (estrogen or glycogen) for the bacteria already present, whereas a probiotic delivers lactobacilli directly to the vagina. It is preferable to deliver these bacteria directly to the vagina using vaginal formulations (suppository or capsule) rather than taking them orally, even one specifically intended for vaginal flora.

Estrogen therapy can be used to treat the vaginal mucosa locally (vaginal cream, suppository) or a hyaluronic acid– or hydrophilic-based gel can be applied three times per week (Replens). Some practitioners also recommend endovaginal laser, which has produced good results.

Anatomy of the Vagina Before and After Menopause

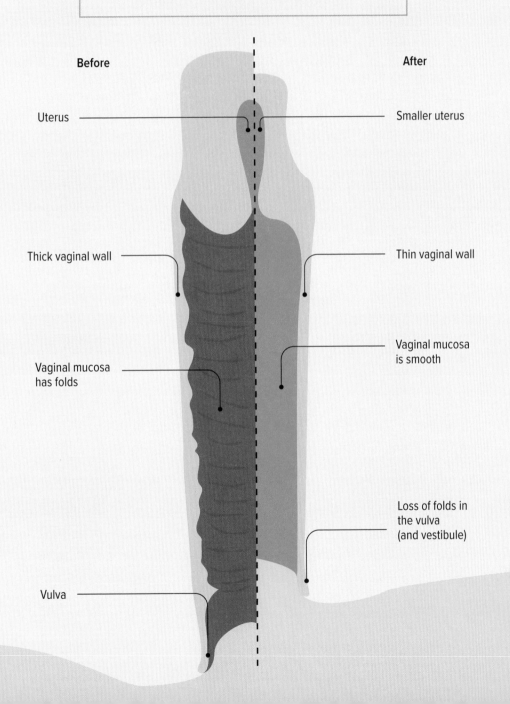

Before

After

Uterus ——————————— Smaller uterus

Thick vaginal wall ————— Thin vaginal wall

Vaginal mucosa
has folds

Vaginal mucosa
is smooth

Loss of folds in
the vulva
(and vestibule)

Vulva —————————

The Vestibule

Estrogen-based cream should be applied one to two times per day for an extended period of time. It's also a good idea to take this opportunity to massage and soften up the tissues. If estrogen is contraindicated, massage this area anyway but with a protective, healing lotion that is vitamin E, hyaluronic acid or zinc oxide based. You can also try Saint-John's-wort or calendula oil. For bathing, use vagina-friendly soaps with an appropriate pH level or emollient. Avoid using sanitary pads and panty liners, which can be irritating and sometimes cause an allergic reaction.

If you have tearing or significant atrophy, an injection of hyaluronic acid can partly revitalize the vestibular and vaginal mucosa. For women who want to do this, the technique can increase the volume of the labia minora, which loses its texture as we age.

▌ Sleep and Mood Problems ▌

When you sleep poorly, you wake up in a bad mood. If you have hot flashes on top of that, you're ready to curse the entire planet! And it's also not easy to keep your spirits up when you add menopause symptoms to the existential questions of midlife! But you'll see, there are always ways to bounce back.

Regain Restorative Sleep

If you have already been experiencing insomnia, you can't blame your sleepless nights on menopause! However, we tend to be lighter sleepers as we age, and when you add hot flashes to the mix, it can mean restless nights. Menopause hormone treatment, particularly progestin, has been shown to be effective for mild sleep problems when taken at night, since it causes drowsiness. In phytotherapy, the winning combination is the trio of lemon balm, valerian and passionflower. Don't give in to the siren call of sleeping pills, since the risk of dependency with benzodiazepines is too great.

> **Don't give in to the siren call of sleeping pills, since the risk of dependency with benzodiazepines is too great.**

The Secrets to a Good Sleep

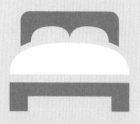

Keep the same routine and know how to identify the signs of fatigue: itchy eyes, yawning...

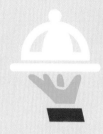

Cut down on fat at meals and limit alcohol intake.

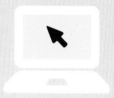

Keep tablets, cell phones and anything with an LED screen out of the bedroom (they decrease melatonin production).

Go to bed and get up at specific times, even if you slept poorly.

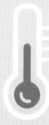

Keep the temperature of your bedroom between 60°F and 70°F (17–20°C).

Make sure it's dark and quiet when you sleep.

ZZZ

Avoid afternoon naps.

Preventing Mood Swings!

Although perimenopause is a time when hormones are all over the place with emotions often changing at the drop of a hat, laughing one minute and tears the next, menopause is a stabilizing period.

According to the Austrian psychoanalyst Hélène Deutsch-Rosenbach (1884–1982), there are two possible paths for women at menopause: wallow in depression or channel all of their creative tendencies toward sublimation. Very harsh!

It's true that we see real cases of post-menopausal depression with no trigger other than the end of menstruation. In this context, hormonal treatment is often a satisfactory solution. There are other specific cases that are much less typical, since we are also dealing with the impact of climacteric symptoms (hot flashes and vaginal dryness topping the list).

And sometimes at 50, we start to question our lives — our relationship as a couple and our families — after the kids have left the nest. And what if this time of deep psychological rethinking is an opportunity to see a therapist?

In terms of phytotherapy, Saint-John's-wort has some anti-depressive properties, but it should be taken with caution, since it can interact with certain drugs. Don't take it without talking to your doctor.

It's no surprise that physical activity has a positive effect on mood, and magnesium and omega-3 can be helpful if you're feeling down.

But you may not need any of this, since, as Hélène Deutsch-Rosenbach indicated with her "sublimation," menopause can be a time when new horizons open up for you to explore: music, painting, writing, spirituality, travel, taking on a humanitarian or charitable cause, or any other passion you may have!

Your Sex and Love Life

▌Everyone Has Their Own Rhythm ▌

Menopause is another step in a woman's life that is a balancing act from one stage to another. Puberty, menstruation, pregnancy and menopause each mark a new beginning. Men have a very different perception of time and its impact. Let's take a moment to understand how menopause can change things in a relationship.

A woman has an internal clock with both cyclical and linear time, marking things that happen before, after, that will never happen again or that are still possible. Menopause can happen suddenly or be a gradual process, upending not only personal and private time but also conjugal and social time, and this affects men as well. Whether she likes it or not, a woman experiences life as a series of befores and afters; a man has a more linear perception of time, and his view is not based on internal markers, as it is for a woman, but external ones. Men tend to be less affected by the passage of time, since their time references are outside their bodies: no periods that come and go and are then gone for good; no uterus with the promise of a new life and then diapers; no breasts that can be nurturing one minute and erotic the next.

For men, time has more of a social context, punctuated by stages of life such as military service (in earlier times) and career progression now. Although men also perceive time in a way that is similar to women — pregnancies, for example — they experience such events somewhat indirectly, since they do not experience them in their own bodies. And don't forget that many couples now go on to successive relationships. This important sociological change has come about over a single generation. This phenomenon is shared equally between women and their partners because they too have sometimes chosen (or experienced) several chapters in their lives.

Men often become aware of the passage of time when their spouse goes through menopause. According to a study conducted in Geneva about difficult life stages, women experience fewer difficult times after age 46, while men can have a major life crisis between the ages of 43 and 52, coinciding with having achieved their goals in terms of social status and a growing awareness of the end of that period of their life.[4] However, at that age, women of that age are at a disadvantage compared to men in terms of the focus placed on youth. Older men are seen as handsome gray foxes, but older women are not necessarily seen in the same way, even though they are in the prime of their life.

> **It's often when their spouses go through menopause that men become aware of the passage of time.**

Yet these women are beautiful and radiant and (hopefully) doing things to stay that way, including getting lots of exercise, eating well, meditating, taking care of their skin and hair, seeking medical care and dressing to suit their style. The purpose of all this is not to deny the passage of time, but instead to embrace new opportunities.

4. E. Perrin and M. Senarclens, "Perspectives socio-psychosomatiques: femmes et ménopause, homme et crise de la cinquantaine," *Méd. Psychosom.*, 1988.

▮ The Female Perspective ▮

Menopause is a great time in a woman's sex life! For the lucky ones: no need to worry about birth control, the kids are settled (hopefully...), a fulfilling career, interesting life experiences and family and friends they can rely on.

In terms of hormones, even though low estrogen dries up the mucosa, the presence of the male hormone testosterone can boost the libido. If your relationship "was working" okay beforehand and if you've already managed to overcome the challenges that life has undoubtedly thrown at you, a short dry spell at the start of menopause will only be a blip.

Sometimes a traumatic event like an illness can suddenly affect your sex life, and you feel like you don't have anything left. You've lost those butterflies in your stomach that made you want to snuggle up with your partner. Again, no need to panic, counselling will get you through.

If, however, it's been quite some time since your sex life has been earth-shattering or if you find yourself counting tiles on the ceiling during sex, or if you are so miserable that your relationship is heading for a breakup, the advice here will likely not be enough. If things are that bad, you will need to work on your issues first.

Tips for Enhancing Your Sexual Appetite!

1 The less you eat, the less you want to eat

Unlike what you might think, the less sex you have, the less you feel like having sex. So it's unrealistic to expect to be suddenly overcome with desire.

2 The appetite returns by eating

You'll need to put the cart before the horse! In other words, even if you're not feeling wild about having sex, run with it. Women often take a bit longer to experience desire, and it kicks in and gains momentum with foreplay.

3 Eating regularly sustains your appetite and helps you digest

After going without sex for a long period of time, the vaginal mucosa becomes more sensitive, and having sex again can cause minor discomfort, like burning or irritation. A lubricant can temporarily help with this. The vagina is the complete opposite of the Energizer bunny: It doesn't keep running if it is *not* used! Having sex at least once a week helps to maintain good vaginal health, keeps the fire burning and helps reduce tension in a relationship. If you didn't reach nirvana this week, no big deal, you can try again next week!

4 Before sitting down to eat, make sure the table looks nice; it will help set the mood

Before you can feel desire, you have to feel desirable. That starts with a good self-image, which you can work on every day through your physical appearance, intelligence and compassion. Some quick and practical advice: After a shower, apply a body lotion with a light or sultry scent, depending on your mood. This intimate contact with your own body will help you feel pretty and sexy, which is important for you to be able to feel desire.

5 What about something to start?

For a man, the time between an initial sexual stimulus (breast, thigh, naughty thought) and an erection is 6 seconds. A woman needs a good 20 minutes to get in the mood and feel amorous. Only after that, and with foreplay, does a woman feel aroused, which triggers lubrication. To produce hormones conducive to intercourse, you can stimulate your skin and erogenous zones by taking a shower or bath with sensual scents and do a full-body skin peel which, as a bonus, will accentuate the pleasant feeling of being caressed. Start stimulating your erogenous zones, breasts and clitoris when you're in the shower. When you're having trouble getting into the mood for sex, you need to prepare physically and mentally to get back in the game.

> Before you can feel desire, you have to feel desirable.

6 Most of all, you need to "want to want it"

Wanting things to change; defusing any conflict with your partner if necessary and seeing them with fresh eyes, not apathy and resentment; finding your partner attractive and desirable and feel desirable yourself — these are avenues you can explore to help you rediscover desire in your relationship. Your best allies are fantasy, as Willy Pasini puts it so nicely, or phantasm, Sigmund Freud's version.[5]

7 Figure out your ideal frequency

What is that exactly? How do you put this in action? There's nothing easier! Mutually agree on a frequency that works for both of you for restarting the engine. The usual frequency is once a week, and more if you both are game. Obviously, you need to find the right time: A quickie in the morning is not always what you feel like, and the evening doesn't always work because you are worn out after a long day at work. Do you know that a woman's libido is at its peak at three in the afternoon?

So all you have to do is take advantage of those glorious afternoon naps on weekends and holidays, especially since this is not your first rodeo together. You know what works...

If these tips seem a little prescriptive, they are more than just formalities. For a bit of background, these are psycho-behavioral sexology techniques that have been validated, tested and approved by 30 years of gynecological consultations.

5. Pasini is an Italian psychiatrist, sexologist and professor of psychiatry and medical psychology at the University of Geneva.

Rediscovering Pleasure!

During menopause, the vaginal mucosa usually reacts more slowly to arousal, causing vaginal dryness and affecting the quality, or even the existence, of your orgasm.

> **Don't be shy about pleasuring yourself, the old-fashioned way or with toys. It's good for you!**

There are many reasons for this, starting with genitourinary syndrome, as explained earlier. Estrogen deficiency is, of course, part of this, as is lack of desire and not enough foreplay. The longer it takes for lubrication to happen, the longer arousal needs to last. Dryness can be particularly unpleasant. You may not feel as wet, or it may take longer to get there. This domino effect makes the problem even worse. Plus, if your partner has been waiting for a while or if he can't maintain an erection like he did 20 years ago, he will want to cut back on foreplay. Start by using a lubricant. Tell your partner that it's like you've changed from gas to diesel, so you need to be warmed up for longer before getting into gear. He should get the idea right away! If you're solo, if your partner has severe erectile disorders or if you just feel like it, don't be shy about pleasuring yourself, the old-fashioned way or with toys. It's good for you. In order to get the most out of your sexuality during menopause, you may find it helpful to have at least a basic understanding of male sexuality during this same stage in life.

The Domino Effect

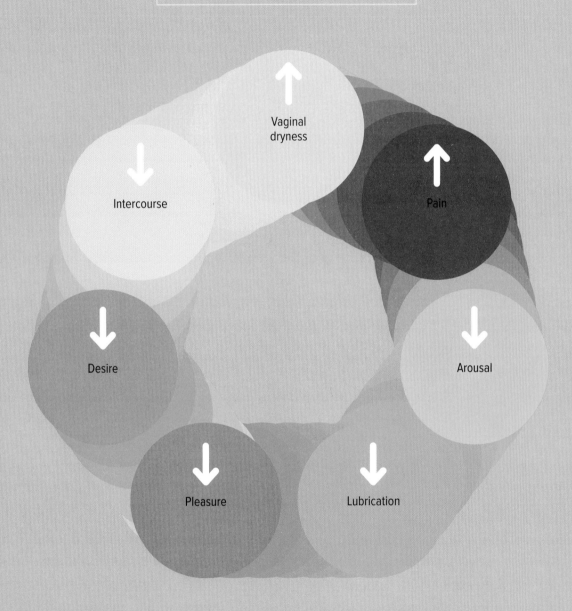

▮ The Male Perspective ▮

Male andropause is not as intense as female menopause. Knowing what lies ahead, women have time to prepare for this particular stage in life, whereas men, who have no idea what is going to happen, may find it more difficult.

Canadian psychologist Yvon Dallaire accurately sums up this stage in life with a bit of humor: "Women fall off a mountain, and men tumble down a hill."[6]

What Happens Around 50 Years of Age?

Around the age of 45 to 50, men's testosterone levels start to decline. It can also occur much later, and not all men are affected. This drop in androgen levels can cause fatigue or depression and a change a man's body: loss of muscle mass, weight gain and even the development of breasts (gynecomastia).

From a sexual perspective, men can experience less desire and also erectile dysfunction. Nothing dramatic in and of itself, since before age 50, one in three men will have experienced impotence, and that number goes up to one in two men after age 50. With age, erectile reactivity decreases. It takes a bit longer to come to attention, and erections don't last as long and aren't as hard.

Nothing to get worked up about, just go with the flow, be playful, don't judge and be reassuring. Reassurance and kindness are key so

6. Y. Dallaire, "L'andropause ou la vie cachée des hommes," *Gérontologie et société*, 2007.

your partner doesn't fall into the downward spiral of fear of failure, which can wreak havoc on a man's ability to maintain an erection!

What Are Their Main Reactions?

When we say that scary word "impotence" (erectile dysfunction is a thousand times better), men usually respond in one of two ways: avoid the problem or take action. When a man avoids the problem, he may choose to limit or deny his desire so he won't be placed in a situation where he can't have an erection. If personal, professional or family problems are also in the picture, a man can experience considerable loss of self-esteem, so the feeling of impotence is not limited to erectile function alone.

From your perspective as a woman, you may feel as though you are no longer desirable, no longer loved. The erectile dysfunction then becomes a relationship problem. My advice is to read this chapter together! Don't be shy to talk about it.

Getting it out in the open is the first thing you should do,

> **After age 50, one in two men will have problems getting an erection.**

and that may be enough to get through this.

When a man responds through action, he may do a variety of things:

• Blame his environment (stress at work, fatigue, sexual or other relationship problems).
• Reassure himself of his "male potency" (seductive or physical) by chasing after younger women or taking on extreme physical activity.
• Decide to deal with it as a couple and, if that does not work, see a specialist.

Of course, the human psyche is much more subtle and complex than what we've discussed here. The objective of this exercise is to see if you can identify anything that resonates with your own situation right now.

Do Erectile Dysfunction Drugs Actually Work?

As long as there is no medical reason for not taking it, that famous little blue pill may save the day. It can show a man that there is nothing wrong with him physically and help him get out of the downward spiral that he's caught up in.

A bit of preplanning, however, is called for. Be supportive and prepared, and the erection may last longer than anticipated.

As well as tablets (such as Viagra, Cialis, Levitra and Stendra), there are two alternative medications, but only one is available in the United States. A man can receive injections at the base of his penis or apply a cream (Vitaros) to the tip of his penis (but FDA approval of the latter is still pending at time of publication). The alternatives to pills are mainly recommended following prostate cancer surgery.

To take the focus off the treatment aspect of things, why not think of this as both of you contributing in an equally important way: you have your lubricant, and he has his Viagra. You each have something to contribute!

The famous little blue pill may help get your partner out of a downward spiral.

▮ We're All in the Same Boat! ▮

After 50, there truly is a parallel between erectile difficulties and vaginal dryness.

Most men and women over 50 have three things in common: biologically, we both experience a drop in sex hormones; sexually, because of how we feel about our ageing bodies, we feel less desirable, so we feel less desire; and lastly, there are major psychological and emotional impacts.

If you had a good sex life before, if you communicate in your relationship and if amorous feelings are not a too-distant memory, this will just be a temporary dry spell. It will get you ready for a new momentum in your sex life — and that's a promise!

Your Body Is Changing

▌ Inside and Out ▌

You can't help but notice that around age 40, or a bit later, there are changes in your figure, weight, skin and hair.

Not everything is hormonal, since some of these changes started long before the period-free year defined as menopause; they can also be attributed to the unstoppable passage of time. So now what? It's not the end of the world. There are certainly enough resources available to help us thumb our noses at time!

The parts of our bodies that are visible are only the tip of the iceberg. Below the surface, our bones, joints, heart and blood vessels are also undergoing changes related to age and meno-pause. Adopting healthy habits and applying sage advice can help mitigate the damage.

The Effects of Menopause on the Body

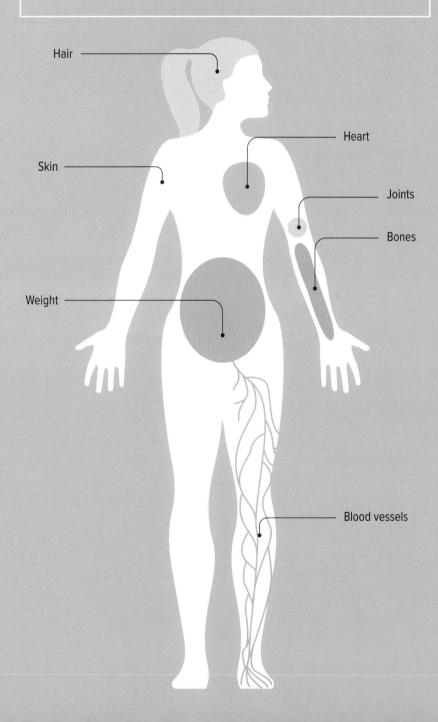

Hair

Skin

Weight

Heart

Joints

Bones

Blood vessels

▎ Your Figure and Weight ▎

You haven't made any major changes in your life, but your clothes just don't fit the way they used to. Things feel tight, especially around the waist.

What's Going On?

This is all due to age-related muscle wasting, a natural process that starts early in life, around age 30, but intensifies once you turn 50.

It all begins with muscle wasting, which begins at 30!

Between the ages of 20 and 70, we lose nearly half of our muscle mass!

Why does this happen? Muscle is constantly changing, with new muscle fibers being produced and older fibers breaking down. This process of metabolism (production) and catabolism (destruction) causes people to gain muscle until about age 30, and then the reverse happens later in life. Two components are needed to produce muscle: physical activity and raw materials, particularly protein. As we age, our visceral organs take in more protein, and less is distributed to muscles. Scientists call this protein retention "splanchnic sequestration."

Eating habits also change over time: Instead of scarfing down prime rib with friends like you did in your 20s, you're having tea and cake! Physical activity is needed to produce muscle, but we become less active with age, so muscle strength decreases.

One last detail, but a weighty one! A person's muscle mass burns 85 percent of their calories, even at rest. That is why when we lose muscle, we gain weight. During this time, our bodies keep chugging away, transforming sugars and other carbs into fat. We have more fat overall, and it's distributed differently. The upper body is less developed, and fat tends to gather in the area between the belly button and knees, especially the belly. Farewell to our slim waist of days gone by! Sometimes, fat settles in the breasts, and we find ourselves moving up a bra size!

Less muscle strength, particularly the muscles in the abdomen, spine, and psoas (the muscles connecting the pelvis and femur to the lumbar vertebrae, straightening the pelvis) results in changes to your posture:

Your lumbar curve is accentuated, your shoulders slide forward, your pelvis tucks back and your belly protrudes. To maintain a graceful look, you need to untuck your pelvis, tilt it forward and suck in your gut. In other words, you need to lengthen your spine, between your tailbone and the crown of your head, bringing your pubic bone forward and expanding your chest, standing tall. Once you've got this under control,

> **Stretching, Pilates and yoga can work miracles for your posture.**

you need to keep focusing on proper posture to correct it, until it becomes natural.

Stretches, Hypopressive exercises, Pilates and the trio of tai chi, qigong and yoga can work miracles for your posture.

Beware of Bad Posture!

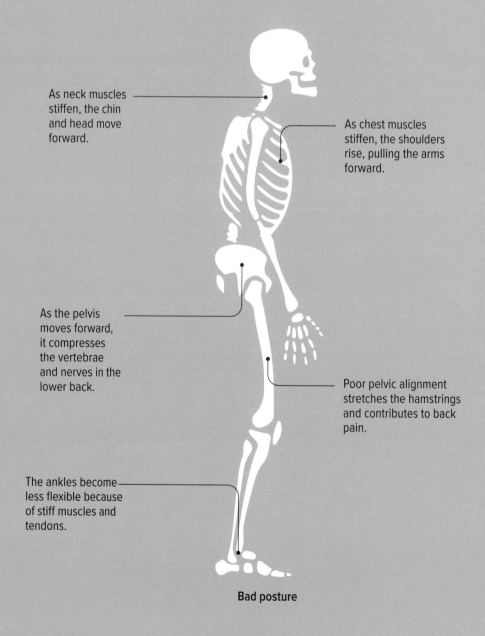

As neck muscles stiffen, the chin and head move forward.

As chest muscles stiffen, the shoulders rise, pulling the arms forward.

As the pelvis moves forward, it compresses the vertebrae and nerves in the lower back.

Poor pelvic alignment stretches the hamstrings and contributes to back pain.

The ankles become less flexible because of stiff muscles and tendons.

Bad posture

How Can You Adopt Good Posture?

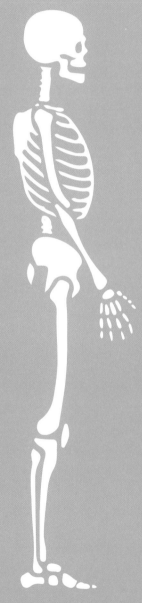

For ideal posture, keep your head in line with your pelvis, your shoulders back and your back straight.

Ideal posture

How Can You Slow Down Muscle Loss?

The answer is fairly simple once you understand how everything works: Increase your dietary intake of protein and exercise more. The recommended daily intake of protein for an adult woman is 0.8 grams/kilogram of body weight (to convert your weight from pounds to kilograms, simply multiply it by 0.36). The recommended amount of protein generally increases with age to 1 gram/kilogram of body weight. Women who are very active should aim for 1.2 grams of protein per kilogram.

Change Your Eating Habits

There are a multitude of diets, each claiming to be the one, the only, the best! Keep in mind that you will always have to compromise. For example, animal protein is excellent for your muscles but not great for your blood vessels. However, everyone agrees on one thing: simple carbs are your worst enemy. Whenever possible, avoid sugary foods, which is obvious! But you also need to stay away from potatoes, white bread, white flour and pasta. Instead, choose complex carbs, including whole-grain pasta and bread and brown rice. There's nothing to stop you from having a little apple pie now and then, as long as you have it after a complete meal that also contains fiber and protein. Eat fruit at mealtimes rather than during the day.

Choose Your Proteins Wisely

Yes, meat is a natural source of protein, but it should be consumed in limited amounts because it also contains bad fats, which are harmful for your heart and blood vessels. And wouldn't it be reasonable to think about the ethical and ecological issues related to meat production? Fatty fish, like salmon, are a good source of protein, iodine and good fats (omega-3s). Unfortunately, the larger the fish, the higher it is on the food chain, so the higher its levels of mercury and hormones. You should not eat fatty fish more than twice per week. However, white fish is fine, like cod, as well as small fatty fish like sardines, mackerel and herring.

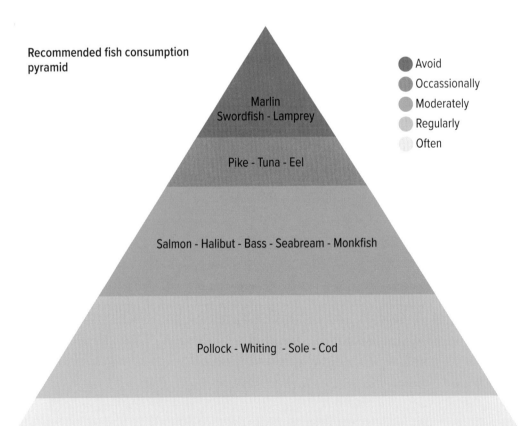

Recommended fish consumption pyramid

Avoid
Occassionally
Moderately
Regularly
Often

Marlin
Swordfish - Lamprey

Pike - Tuna - Eel

Salmon - Halibut - Bass - Seabream - Monkfish

Pollock - Whiting - Sole - Cod

Sardine - Trout - Herring - Mackerel

Dairy products are another way to get your protein, but they also contain saturated animal fat. They do, however, provide the calcium needed for good bone health. Again, everything in moderation. Opt for goat cheese instead of creamy desserts or sugary yogurts, but don't forget about eggs!

A boiled egg for breakfast is great and doesn't increase your cholesterol!!

Did you know that you can eat a boiled egg every day without increasing your cholesterol intake as long as the yolk is soft or runny? When you buy organic eggs, from chickens raised outdoors and fed things like flaxseed, your eggs are a great source of omega-3s. A boiled egg at breakfast is a great way to start the day, and it helps to maintain muscle mass.

So what about plant-based proteins? They're also a very good source of protein. Although vegetarian proteins are less concentrated than meat proteins, they do provide you with vitamins and micronutrients. If you haven't done this already, now might be the time to change your eating habits by introducing chickpeas, quinoa, lentils and split peas to your diet. As mentioned earlier, it's important to keep soy consumption in balance, since a single soy dessert can contain the 45 mg per day that typifies the Asian diet. You can also consider protein shakes, powders and smoothies, which are a great way to top up your breakfast.

Choose the Physical Activity That's Right for You

The best physical activity is something you'll enjoy doing regularly. There are so many options available, you are sure to find something that works with your interests, physical ability, schedule and finances. For the price of a pair of running shoes, you can put a lot of ground behind you by walking, and for the price of a swimsuit you can swim hundreds of laps! You may want to give Nordic walking a try. It's safe and suitable for all ages because the poles prevent falls and help you work your upper body, using 30 percent more energy than simply walking without poles.

All sorts of terrains are suitable, urban or natural. And gyms, of course, offer the latest exercise trends.

There are so many options. Just stay within your physical limitations. However, the more you work out, the more you'll be able to do.

> Why not give Nordic walking a try? It's safe, easy, effective and suitable for everyone!

If exercise is hard-wired in your DNA and you regularly do physical activity, the best advice is: once you turn 50, check in with your doctor and consider a stress test. Don't overdo it, and adapt your workout to your current physical condition. Exercise that includes endurance (medium but continuous exertion) is great, but you should also include a little resistance training (significant exertion in short bursts). To increase your muscle strength, isometric exercises (using static resistance) will promote your muscle development. Furthermore, by adding light weights, your muscles will work harder and you will also strengthen your bones.

Use light weights to make your muscles work harder and strengthen your bones.

Tips for Getting Back into Exercise

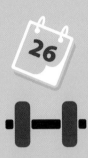

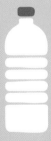

Start slowly and exercise at least 3 times per week for an hour. You will definitely see results.

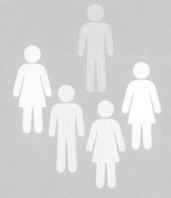

Exercise with others to help you stay motivated.

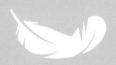

Take care of your joints: no sharp movements or stretching beyond what is comfortable.

Don't forget to hydrate after exercise and to incorporate protein in your diet.

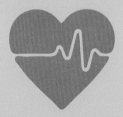

Talk to your doctor if you have a heart condition or if your workout requires considerable physical exertion.

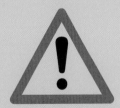

If you have confirmed osteoporosis, think carefully about sports with a risk of falling, such as cycling, skiing and horseback riding.

If you're starting from scratch because exercise has never been a regular part of your life, it's not too late to get moving! Slow and steady are what you need to remember and put into action.

It's never too late to start exercising!

Ideally, you should follow an exercise program that is supervised by a professional.

Some physiotherapy offices offer group exercise classes that you can take advantage of: It's often cheaper than a gym membership. Based on what you learn, you can put together your own 15-minute morning wake-up workout, which will get you ready to face the day.

Many thanks to Dr. Guillaume Muff for his valuable advice and help writing this chapter.

Get the Most out of Your Day

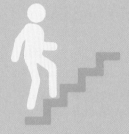

Don't take the elevator if you're only going up or down four flights of stairs or less.

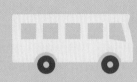

Don't take the bus or subway when you're only going a few stops, and get off one stop early, if possible.

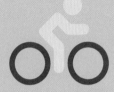

Hop on your bike for intermediate distances that are too far to walk.

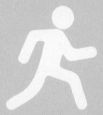

Do your errands on foot in your neighborhood.

Jump up any time anybody asks for the salt, a pen, a coffee, etc.

Live the adage "Even if you've lost your head, you've still got your legs," and retrace your steps when you forget something.

When on vacation, go for a walk or swim instead of lounging poolside.

▪ Your Bones and Joints ▪

Our bones and joints start to decline with age, and menopause is a definite (and often painful) turning point.

As we age, we lose bone mass and our joints decline and aren't as flexible. Why is that? Simply because estrogen is vital for calcium to bind to bone and is part of bone anabolism (the production of new bone). Joints have estrogen receptors. When there is an estrogen deficiency, joints can become painful and less flexible, especially first thing in the morning, which is why it can take a bit of effort to roll yourself out of bed in the morning.

Your Joints

When there is an estrogen deficiency, joints become painful and less flexible overall. However, what is most painful is osteoarthritis, which actually has nothing to do with your hormones. Instead, it's caused by wear and tear of the cartilage, like that good old osteoarthritis of the hip, which causes so many hip replacements! Osteoporosis and osteoarthritis are often confused. Osteoporosis is when there is bone loss. It is not painful, unless it leads to a fracture or vertebral compression. Osteoarthritis is when there is excess bone development, especially around the joints. In vertebrae, these bone spurs or osteophytes can take the shape of parrots' beaks along the spine.

Changes in Bone Mass Over Time

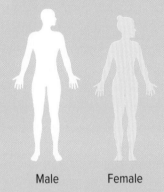

Male   Female

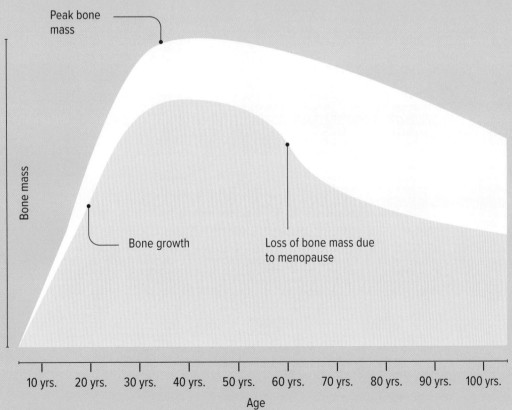

Peak bone mass

Bone growth

Loss of bone mass due to menopause

Bone mass

10 yrs.   20 yrs.   30 yrs.   40 yrs.   50 yrs.   60 yrs.   70 yrs.   80 yrs.   90 yrs.   100 yrs.

Age

Bone Mass

How Does Bone Mass Develop and Change?

Bone mass starts to form at birth, peaks around age 30, plateaus and then decreases gradually and more sharply at menopause. The main factors for individual variation in bone mass are:

- genetics;
- sex (advantage men!);
- age;
- diet, particularly calcium and vitamin D intake;
- physical activity.

How Is Bone Mass Measured?

Bone mineral density (BMD) is measured using a digital X-ray technique. Although it would seem logical for there to be a connection between density and solidity, this exam alone cannot predict the risk of fracture with any certainty, hence, the need for preventive treatment.

Another approach consists of measuring biochemical bone resorption markers through a C-terminal cross-linked telopeptide (CTX) test. High levels indicate active bone loss. The best way to identify whether you are at risk for osteoporosis is to stay on top of your medical history.

The risk factors indicating that BMD should be measured are:
- personal history of fracture following a moderate impact;
- first-degree family history (father or mother) of hip fracture;
- thin build with a body mass index below 19;
- long-term cortisone therapy (to treat asthma or rheumatoid arthritis, for example);
- any hormonal fluctuations involving an estrogen deficiency for an extended period of time, such as early menopause, anorexia nervosa or treatment with aromatases inhibitors;
- smoking.

The result of this exam, performed at two sites, the spine and femur, is plotted on a curve according to age: measurement may be normal, osteopenic (BMD is low but not pathological) or pathological, indicating osteoporosis.

Osteoporosis

What Exactly Is It?

Osteoporosis is a bone disease in which bones become more fragile due to decreased mineral density as well as bone remodeling. Osteoporosis leads to an increased risk of fracture from minor trauma. The most characteristic fractures are of the wrist, hip and vertebrae, also called vertebral compression. In the United States, around half of all women aged 50 and older will break a bone due to osteoporosis. Across the country, osteoporosis is the cause of some 2 million broken bones annually, resulting in $19 billion in related costs. Meanwhile, in Canada,

> The best way to determine if you are at risk for osteoporosis is staying on top of your medical history.

80 percent of all fractures in menopausal women aged 50 and older are caused by osteoporosis. Moreover, one in three hip fracture patients will re-fracture within a year, and 28 percent of women who suffer a hip fracture will die within a year. These numbers, which are quite concerning, show the importance of being proactive, which is entirely possible!

Osteoporosis

40 years	60 years	70 years

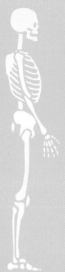
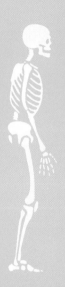
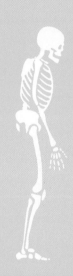

Normal tight bone material with good calcification = solid bone

Bone mass reduced; bone material looser and less dense

Osteoporosis; bone material very reduced; poor calcification; multiple cavities = fragile bone

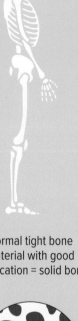
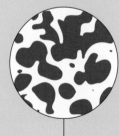
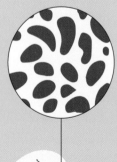
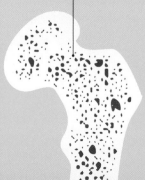
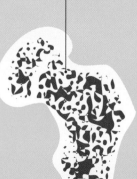
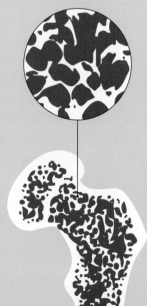

How Can You Prevent Osteoporosis?

Even though you can't change your genetics, you still have control over your diet, which needs to be balanced and include a sufficient intake of calcium and vitamin D, which are your bones' best friends.

Calcium

A menopausal woman needs 1,200 mg of calcium per day. The best sources of calcium in food are milk and other dairy products. If you do not consume these, you can opt for a calcium-fortified mineral water or other calcium-fortified non-dairy beverage. Many foods are also a good source of calcium, such as sardines, anchovies, herring, eggs and some plants (to find out more about these plant-based calcium sources, see the following pages).

Dairy Products

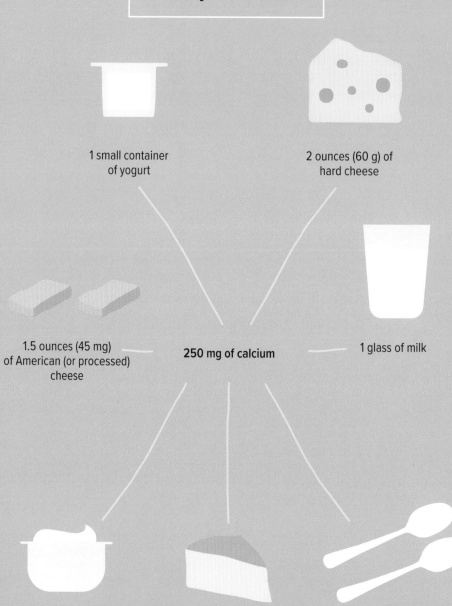

1 small container
of yogurt

2 ounces (60 g) of
hard cheese

1.5 ounces (45 mg)
of American (or processed)
cheese

250 mg of calcium

1 glass of milk

1 cup (250 ml) of plain Greek
yogurt

2 ounces (60 g) of soft cheese

2 tablespoons of powdered
skim milk

Vegan Products

Hazelnuts (4.5 ounces / 125 g)

Parsley (4.5 ounces / 125 g)

Chickpeas (7 ounces / 190 g)

Corn salad or mâche (9 ounces / 250 g)

Basil (4.5 ounces / 125 g)

Sesame seeds (1 ounce / 30 g)

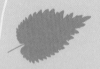

Nettles (1.25 ounces / 35 g)

Green cabbage (11 ounces / 310 g)

250 mg of calcium

White beans (6 ounces / 175 g)

Almonds (3.5 ounces / 100 g)

Dried figs (4.5 ounces / 130 g)

Arugula (5.5 ounces / 155 g)

Broccoli (9 ounces / 250 g)

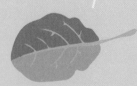

Spinach (3 ounces / 90 g)

Fennel (9 ounces / 250 g)

Dandelion (5.25 ounces / 150 g)

Vitamin D

Did you know that in the United States, 50 to 60 percent of nursing home residents and hospitalized patients have a vitamin D deficiency? And did you know that in Canada, about 25 percent of the population has an insufficient level of vitamin D during the summer, but that number rises to 40 percent during the winter?

> 50 to 60 percent of nursing home residents have a vitamin D deficiency.

Without this important vitamin, calcium is poorly absorbed in the intestines; it leaks into the urine and doesn't bind to bone. The recommended daily intake of vitamin D for a woman over 50 is 15 micrograms or 600 IU (international units). However, dietary intake is rarely sufficient. The sun also plays a very important role.

Our skin is able to synthesize vitamin D from sunlight, provided our body can be exposed to the sun for 15 minutes. Therefore, regular supplementation is critical for nearly everyone, and even more important for menopausal women. Discuss vitamin D with your health-care provider and find out if you can obtain a prescription. The only proven benefits of vitamin D are for bones, but many studies suggest it has other positive effects as well and can help prevent certain cancers (breast, colon, prostate and pancreas), reduce cardiovascular risk and provide immune and infectious defenses. In short, vitamin D does just about everything except the dishes!

Exercises to Help Prevent Osteoporosis

Movements that put stress on your bones stimulate bone formation. Therefore exercises involving weights (a bottle of water in each hand will do the trick) or resistance (such as using exercise bands) are recommended. When walking, consider using poles, which provides benefits for your arm bones, particularly your wrist bones. And wear a small backpack, properly adjusted so your back is straight; it will help you strengthen your femoral neck.

The Power Plate platform and similar devices can also be effective. They can often be found at occupational therapy centers and gyms, or you can purchase one and use it at home.

By stimulating calcium to bind to bone, physical activity helps prevent osteoporosis.

Treatments

Treatments can be divided into three categories: bisphosphonates, SERMs (selective estrogen receptor modifiers) and — menopausal hormone therapy!

There are various types of osteoporosis treatments. Talk to your doctor to find out more.

The treatment that's best for you depends on your age, the primary site of your osteoporosis (vertebrae or hip), your own contraindications and whether you want to take advantage of the other effects of hormonal treatment for hot flashes and vaginal dryness, for example. In short, to find out what treatment is best for you, talk to your health-care provider.

How to Keep Osteoporosis at Bay

Have solid, well-calcified bones when you reach menopause.

Make sure you get enough calcium and vitamin D.

Don't smoke and cut back on alcohol.

Be as active as possible and exercise regularly.

Maintain a healthy weight and treat any hormonal amenorrhea.

▮ Your Heart and Blood Vessels ▮

The cardiovascular system isn't happy about the deficiency in natural estrogen either, and we know that there is a higher risk for heart disease after menopause.

Estrogen supports both the vascular endothelium (the lining inside blood vessels), and it helps prevent atherosclerosis (the loss of elasticity in the arteries). Estrogen also improves your fat (lipid) profile, particularly the ratio between "good" and "bad" cholesterol. We

Cardiovascular risk is higher after menopause: be advised!

know that cardiovascular risk is higher after menopause. Atherosclerosis can lead to heart attacks and stroke: fat deposits accumulate on the walls of blood vessels, causing them to narrow and the deposits sometimes detach, blocking a smaller blood vessel further along.

This is not a reason to sit back and do nothing; there are things you can do! If you are at risk (family or personal history of cardiovascular disease, obesity, high blood pressure, diabetes, high cholesterol, smoking), discuss your health with your doctor.

Regardless of your medical history, make sure you eat a healthy, balanced diet and exercise regularly. Do go easy on the dairy products if you have high "bad" cholesterol. Don't just rely on your total cholesterol, since the risk of high cholesterol is based on the ratio between "good" cholesterol (HDL) and "bad" cholesterol (LDL).

Good fats can be found in fish, olive oil, canola oil and nuts. Bad cholesterol is found in animal fats (dairy products, fatty meat, cold cuts) and saturated oils (sunflower, peanut and palm).

▮ Your Skin, Hair and Nails ▮

Your skin is your primary contact with your environment. How it looks is a reflection of your health and vitality. Epithelial appendages, a scientific word that simply refers to hair and nails, are also parts of yourself that you need to take care of.

Your Skin

Estrogen deficiency (yet again!) makes our skin thinner and more fragile as we age, and there is less connective tissue, which provides support. Wrinkles form and features begin to sag. Maintaining good skin depends on a number of factors: age (of course), lifestyle, genetics and menopause. You can't rely solely on your age or genetics however.

At menopause, even hormonal treatment cannot guarantee you have baby-smooth skin until you're 70. Focus on maintaining good lifestyle habits and keep smiling! After all, there is an undeniable charm and beauty to a face with expression lines that reflect a life full of smiles, just as wrinkles reflect overcoming those more difficult times.

How to Naturally Maintain Glowing Skin

Your real enemies are, unsurprisingly, smoking and sun exposure. If you haven't already done so, it is high time you get help to give up smoking. You should also protect yourself from the sun as much as possible: use sunblock, wear a hat and stick to shade when lounging on a patio, at the beach or anywhere else. Remember to also drink plenty of water; lack of proper hydration can quickly be seen in the skin.

Don't let your skin get dry. Be kind to your skin by using a product that best suits your skin type, never go to bed without completely removing your makeup, thoroughly clean your skin, exfoliate to remove dead cells on the surface with a gentle peel and treat yourself to a hydrating mask every now and then. Ask a dermatologist for advice if you're not sure which products will work best for you.

How to Care for Your Skin

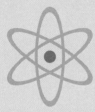

Watch for hormonal changes.

Give yourself an anti-aging massage.

Use ultra-moisturizing creams and lotions.

Remember to apply cream to your hands and neck too.

Don't forget to apply sunscreen.

Drink plenty of water, stay active and eat a healthy diet.

Cosmetic Dermatology and Plastic Surgery

For women who want to and can afford it, cheating a bit is nothing to be embarrassed about. Techniques have evolved a lot since Botox and injections of hyaluronic acid. But let's not be too hasty about putting both products in the Museum of Cosmetic Surgery; they're still very useful in many situations. An injection of hyaluronic acid under the skin helps give the underlying connective tissue more volume and pep to fill in a wrinkle or an area of the face where lines are starting to form.

The real revolution involves physical techniques: laser, radio frequency and pulsed light.

They can help smooth out the complexion and tighten up the skin. A good cosmetic dermatologist should be able to suggest several techniques after a detailed diagnosis of your skin and cosmetic goals.

Cosmetic surgery is more extensive, more costly and sometimes, well, a little much, especially in the cheekbone area, don't you think? On the other hand, if you really don't like what you see in the mirror, there are options you might want to consider. Just do your research and find a certified cosmetic surgeon.

Your Hair

With age and menopause, hair gets thinner and finer. There is a bit of an exception for women who already have very fine hair: As it grays, hair may change and become less straight and get thicker. In terms of the amount of hair, it doesn't grow back like it used to and nothing is guaranteed. There will certainly be less volume. No need to panic! As with the skin, you can do things for your hair. Nutritional supplements can help by providing the constituents of keratin and stimulating regrowth. The main ones are B vitamins, zinc and two amino acids, cysteine and methionine. Zinc may sometimes cause minor digestive disorders and a metallic taste in the mouth.

If you have any androgenic hair loss (at your temples and top of your head), talk to a dermatologist. Most women, fortunately, do not have any underlying medical

Vitamin B, zinc, cysteine and methionine help strengthen hair.

conditions that affect their hair, so all you likely need to do is pamper your hair with a gentle shampoo, volumizing products and a hair mask every now and then. Maybe it's also a good time to try out a new hairstyle?

Menopausal Hormone Therapy

What can you expect from menopausal hormone therapy (MHT)?

Well, it's quite simple: no more hot flashes, the vaginal mucosa of a young woman (or close enough), improved sleep (mainly because those nighttime hot flashes go away), fewer mood swings, better muscle tone, more solid bones, a sharper mind (improved cognitive function in medical jargon) and less hardening of blood vessels. Not bad, right?

▮ What's All the Fuss About? ▮

In the 2000s, American and English studies showed that when MHT (also called hormone replacement therapy, or HRT) is used, as prescribed in those countries, the risk of breast cancer was 1.6 times higher. However, a French study started in 1990 and still ongoing, with a cohort of 80,000 women, has shown that taking a biologically similar progestin does not significantly increase the risk of breast cancer in the first 5 years of treatment.[7]

7. Jacques E. Rossouw et al., "Risks and Benefits of Estrogen Plus Progestin in Healthy Postmenopausal Women: Principal Results from the Women's Health Initiative Randomized Controlled Trial", *JAMA* 288, no. 3 (July 17, 2002): 321–33; "Breast Cancer and Hormone Replacement Therapy: Collaborative Reanalysis of Data from 51 Epidemiological Studies of 52,705 Women with Breast Cancer and 108,411 Women Without Breast Cancer", Lancet 350, no. 9084 (October 11, 1997): 1047–59; Agnès Fournier et al., "Unequal Risks for Breast Cancer Associated with Different Hormone Replacement Therapies : Results from the E3N Cohort Study," *Breast Cancer Research and Treatment* 107, no. 1 (January 2008): 103–11.

After that, the risk is 1.2 times higher, quickly returning to normal when treatment is stopped. In that study, the annual incidence rate of breast cancer rose from 94.7 women out of 100,000 to 113.7 out of 100,000 after 5 years of MHT, meaning about 2 additional breast cancers per 10,000 women per year.

Due to the potential risks involved, the FDA recommends that MHT always be prescribed at the lowest effective dose and only for as long as needed. MHT is also sometimes recommended for prevention of postmenopausal osteoporosis, if bone-specific treatment is not possible.

Surprisingly, a drop in the risk of colon cancer has been observed in MHT users, although there is no explanation for this usual finding.

The other concern related to MHT use is cardiovascular risk. The same American and English studies did show an increase in stroke and heart attack.

> The risks and benefits of MHT should be reassessed each year.

Newer studies clearly show that the use of transdermal natural estrogen (estradiol in the form of a gel or patch) actually decrease the risk of cardiovascular disease.[8] This is logical, since estrogen has a protective effect on the cardiovascular system, particularly related to arterial risks (stroke and heart attack). In terms of venous risks (phlebitis and pulmonary embolisms), it's more controversial, since results depend on the type of estrogen and how it is administered. However, a French study showed that if the natural hormone is administered transdermally, there's no increased risk for venous thromboembolic events.[9]

With these scientific references, you now have everything you need to respond to the naysayers who want to scare you off MHT!

To put it simply, if you don't have any contraindications (breast or uterine cancer, history of phlebitis, family risk of phlebitis or embolism) and are finding menopause difficult, you may want to consider MHT and then see for yourself how it works!

8. Christel Renoux et al., "Transdermal and Oral Hormone Replacement Therapy and the Risk of Stroke: A Nested Case-Control Study," *BMJ* 340 (2010): c2519.

9. Pierre-Yves Scarabin et al., "Differential Association of Oral and Transdermal Oestrogen-Replacement Therapy with Venous Thromboembolism Risk," *Lancet* 362, no. 9362 (August 9, 2003): 428–32.

▌ So Really, What Should I Do? ▌

If you want to start MHT, you still need to wait for menopause to be confirmed by waiting out one year without any periods.

In most cases, MHT combines two hormones: estrogen (I recommend transdermal estradiol in gel or patch form) and progestin. There are also pills that combine the two hormones, but the progestin in those products is not biologically similar to natural progesterone, and they also necessitate that the estrogen be taken orally.

Let's explore estrogen first, since it's the hormone that's really life-altering when it comes to menopausal symptoms. This is because the problems you experience during menopause are caused by estrogen deficiency.

Estrogen should ideally be administered transdermally (i.e., through the skin). Several forms are available, including patches, gels, creams, sprays and vaginal rings. Ideally, the gel or cream should be applied after showering, over a large area of the thigh or belly but absolutely not on the breasts. It should be rubbed in until it is absorbed by the skin.

Since the goal is to find the minimum effective dose, I prefer the gel since it's the easiest to adjust. For example, you could start with two pumps per day, but if you're

> In MHT, estrogen should ideally be applied transdermally (though the skin).

still getting hot flashes after two weeks, your health-care provider can increase your dose to three pumps per day. If, however, your breasts are tender, this indicates that the dose is too high, so you can then decrease your dose by one pump per day. Easy, right? You and your doctor can easily control the treatment!

In MHT, progestin is only used to protect the lining of the uterus (endometrium) from estrogen. In the absence of progestin, there is a risk of uterine cancer. Progestin should be taken at bedtime, since it causes drowsiness (great for those who have trouble sleeping) and dizziness. The progestin capsule may also be placed directly inside your vagina. In this case, the progestin does not cause any dizziness or drowsiness but still protects the endometrium.

If you've had a hysterectomy, you don't have a uterus or endometrium, so there's no need for progestin.

In practice, after 5 years of treatment, it's a good idea to consider the advisability of continuing. A therapeutic window (stopping treatment temporarily) is all that's needed to see how you feel without MHT. Most often, women do not last more than a month off their MHT, as all of the problems that justified the treatment come roaring back, with hot flashes leading the charge. On the other hand, it might be beneficial to very gradually lower the dose of estrogen to try to reach the minimum dose that provides a good quality of life. Over the years, you'll find you need less and less!

> In MHT, progestin is only used to protect the lining of the uterus from estrogen.

To stay "meno-optimistic," repeat the 10 commandments of the menopausal woman to yourself regularly. No big deal! Dealing with menopause and getting through it smoothly requires, first of all, the right state of mind. Honestly, what bothers you most? The physical discomforts or getting older? What other people think or what you think? I'm just asking you to look at it all a bit differently!

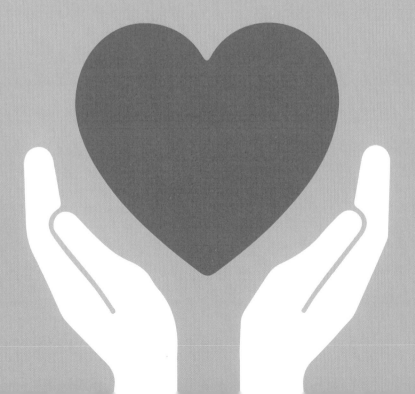

The 10 Commandments for Menopausal Women

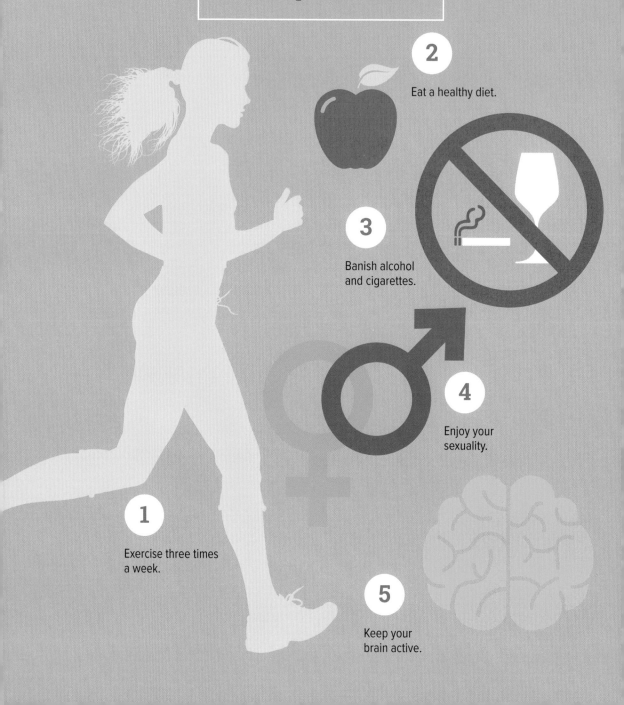

2 Eat a healthy diet.

3 Banish alcohol and cigarettes.

4 Enjoy your sexuality.

1 Exercise three times a week.

5 Keep your brain active.

6

Take time to meditate and reduce stress.

7

Develop your relationships.

8

Take care of your appearance.

9

Take time out for yourself and real vacations.

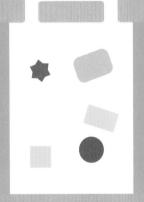

10

Be kind to yourself.

Conclusion

Menopause is not a time in a woman's life when things wrap up and come to an end. Instead, it is a time for new beginnings and a fresh start. Up to now, we've been listening to that constant "tick, tock, tick, tock" of our biological clock. We've fearlessly taken on the challenges of family life (and reaped the rewards) and struggled for fair treatment at work. Now it's finally time to focus on ourselves! This does not mean morphing into a self-absorbed ego-maniac. Instead, we need to think of this as a time to catch up on interests we may have set aside for many years and approach this task with enthusiasm and no hidden agenda! We know our value and our limitations and that we have choices, so now we need to explore our full potential! We are empowered women after all, right? Although everything's not perfect — we don't have the body of our youth and may have experienced illness or loneliness — we need to be kind to ourselves and focus on what's inside and not obsess about an increasing waistline. I wish you all the best on your journey!

Index

Numbers in bold indicate an illustration.

Table of Illustrations

The author

Odile Bagot is a gynecologist and obstetrician with a degree in psychosomatic gynecology. She has been in private practice for over 25 years and is a former hospital clinic head. She holds a masters in ethics and teaches sexology at the University of Strasbourg, in France. A contented woman in her 60s, she has gone through and gloriously survived menopause. Through her blog (Mam Gynéco), Facebook page and involvement with various magazines and websites (including Elle), she provides sound medical advice in plain language and a positive way. She is also the author of *Your Vagina: Everything You Need to Know!*

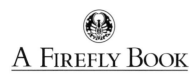

A FIREFLY BOOK

Published by Firefly Books Ltd. 2021
English translation © Firefly Books Ltd. 2021
Text © Odile Bagot 2019
Image Credit: Thinkstockphotos
© First published in French by Mango, Paris, France 2019
as *MÉNOPAUSE: pas de panique !* (9782317019685)

First printing

Library of Congress Control Number: 2020950240

Library and Archives Canada Cataloguing in Publication
Title: Menopause : no need to panic / Odile Bagot, Doctor of Gynecology.
Other titles: Ménopause, pas de panique! English
Names: Bagot, Odile, author.
Description: Translation of: Ménopause, pas de panique! | Includes index.
Identifiers: Canadiana 20200382853 | ISBN 9780228103219 (softcover)
Subjects: LCSH: Menopause—Popular works.
Classification: LCC RG186 .B3413 2021 | DDC 618.1/75—dc23

Published in Canada by
Firefly Books Ltd.
50 Staples Avenue, Unit 1
Richmond Hill, Ontario
L4B 0A7

Published in the United States by
Firefly Books (U.S.) Inc.
P.O. Box 1338, Ellicott Station
Buffalo, New York
14205

Design and Layout: Cyril Terrier
Translator: Priscilla Hendrickson

Printed in China

 Canadä We acknowledge the financial support of the Government of Canada